Routledge Revivals

THE PSYCHOLOGY OF MEDICINE

THE PSYCHOLOGY
OF MEDICINE

BY
T. W. MITCHELL, M.D.

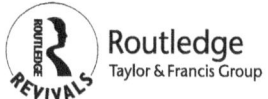

Routledge
Taylor & Francis Group

First published in 1921 by Methuen & Co. Ltd.

This edition first published in 2018 by Routledge
2 Park Square, Milton Park, Abingdon, Oxon, OX14 4RN
and by Routledge
711 Third Avenue, New York, NY 10017

Routledge is an imprint of the Taylor & Francis Group, an informa business

© 1921 Taylor & Francis

Publisher's Note
The publisher has gone to great lengths to ensure the quality of this reprint
but points out that some imperfections in the original copies may be
apparent.

Disclaimer
The publisher has made every effort to trace copyright holders and
welcomes correspondence from those they have been unable to contact.
A Library of Congress record exists under ISBN:

ISBN 13: 978-1-138-55564-8 (hbk)
ISBN 13: 978-1-138-56855-6 (pbk)
ISBN 13: 978-0-203-70505-6 (ebk)

THE PSYCHOLOGY OF MEDICINE

BOOKS ON PSYCHOLOGY

AN INTRODUCTION TO SOCIAL PSYCHOLOGY.
By Professor WILLIAM McDOUGALL, F.R.S. Sixteenth Edition. Crown 8vo. 8s. 6d. net.

BODY AND MIND : A History and a Defence of Animism. By WILLIAM McDOUGALL, F.R.S. With 13 Diagrams. Fifth Edition. Demy 8vo. 12s. 6d. net.

NATIONAL WELFARE AND NATIONAL DECAY.
By WILLIAM McDOUGALL, F.R.S., Professor of Psychology at Harvard University. Crown 8vo. 6s. net.

PSYCHOLOGY. A Short Account of the Human Mind. By F. S. GRANGER, M.A., D.Litt., (Lond.) Fourth Edition. Crown 8vo. 5s. net.

AN INTRODUCTION TO PSYCHOLOGY. By S. S. BRIERLEY, M.A. Crown 8vo. 5s. net.

THE PSYCHOLOGY OF SOCIETY. By MORRIS GINSBERG, M.A., Lecturer in Philosophy at University College, London. Crown 8vo. 5s. net.

THE PSYCHOLOGY OF EVERYDAY LIFE. By JAMES DREVER, M.A., B.Sc., D.Phil. Second Edition. Crown 8vo. 6s. net.

THE PSYCHOLOGY OF INDUSTRY. By JAMES DREVER, M.A., B.Sc., D.Phil. Crown 8vo. 5s. net.

THE PSYCHOLOGY OF PERSUASION. By WILLIAM MACPHERSON, M.A. Crown 8vo. 6s. net.

PSYCHO-ANALYSIS. By R. H. HINGLEY, B.A. Crown 8vo. 6s. net.

PSYCHOLOGY AND FOLKLORE. By R. R. MARETT, M.A., D.Sc. Crown 8vo. 7s. 6d. net.

THE PSYCHOLOGY
OF MEDICINE

BY

T. W. MITCHELL, M.D.

METHUEN & CO. LTD.
36 ESSEX STREET W.C.
LONDON

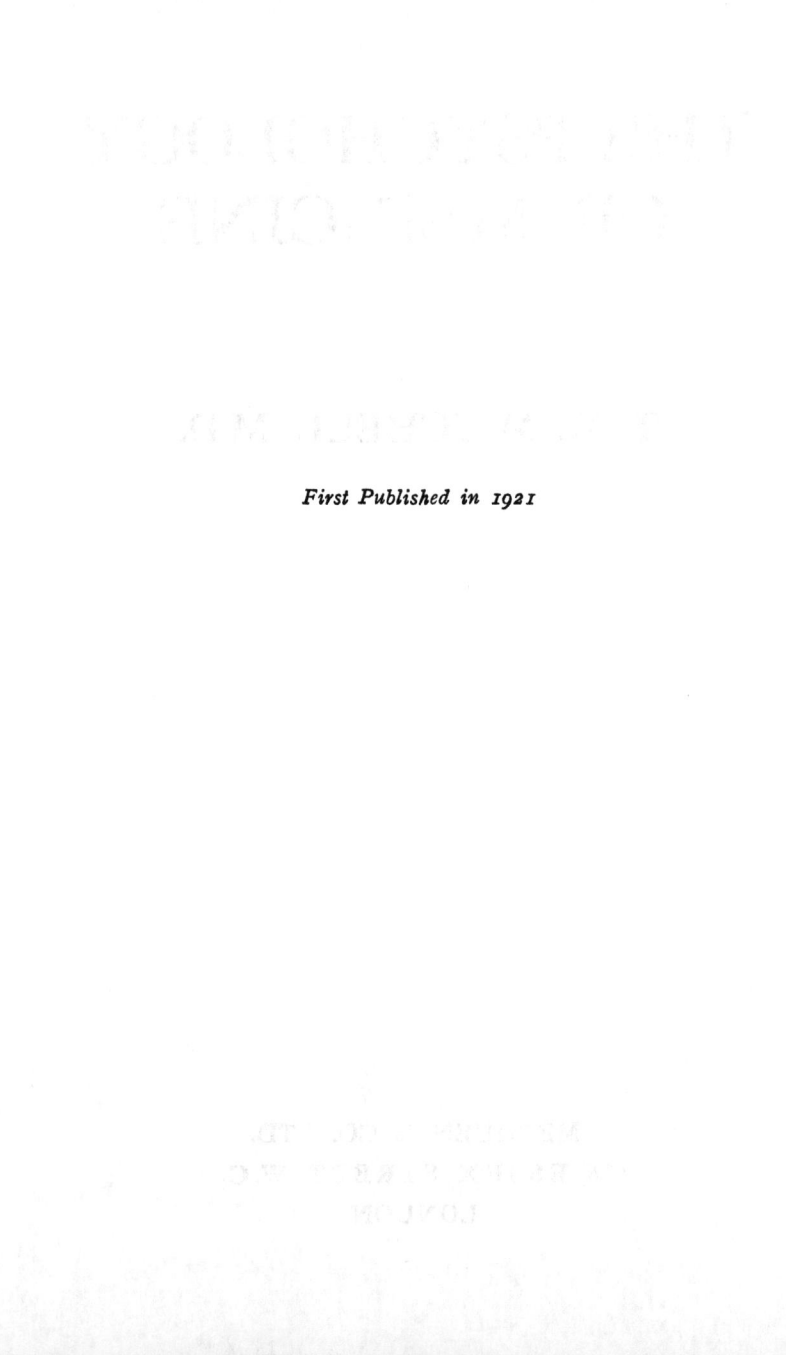

First Published in 1921

PREFACE

THIS book is intended primarily for those readers who have had no professional training in either Medicine or Psychology, but who are anxious to keep themselves abreast of modern thought in these departments of knowledge. At the same time I hope it may prove serviceable to professional students of these subjects as a preliminary survey of the ground they will have to cover should they desire to specialize in psychotherapeutics or in the psychology of the abnormal.

The topics discussed have been dealt with only in outline. My endeavour has been to state the general principles on which modern conceptions in the Psychology of Medicine are based, and to avoid as far as possible all detail which is unnecessary for the comprehension of these principles.

The greater part of the contents is now published for the first time ; but Chapter IV, on " The Unconscious," was largely drawn upon in a paper entitled " Psychology and the Unconscious," read before the Medical Section of the British Psychological Society and published in the *British Journal of Psychology* (Medical Section), Vol. I, Parts 3 and 4, July, 1921. Various paragraphs in the earlier chapters have appeared in articles contributed to the *Proceedings of the Society for Psychical*

Research.   I desire to express my thanks to the Councils of these Societies for permission to make use of these contributions.

My grateful thanks are due to Miss Elsie L. Reynolds for much assistance in preparing the book for the press.

T. W. M.

HADLOW,
    KENT.
        October, 1921.

CONTENTS

THE PSYCHOLOGY OF MEDICINE

CHAPTER I

INTRODUCTION

WE use the word Medicine in a broad sense as a term which includes everything pertaining to the science and art of healing. The practice of medicine is the making use of all and every means whereby those who are sick in body or in mind may be restored to health. From the earliest times it was observed that all bodily disease has a mental aspect, such as the subjective experience of pain, of mental depression or of excitement, and that such mental experiences as sorrow or anxiety are accompanied by some loss of bodily well-being.

Although in primitive medicine the interdependence of body and mind was accepted as self-evident truth, and the possibility of mental and occult influences affecting bodily disorders was widely believed in, with the rise of the scientific era men readily inclined to the view that both the cause and the cure of disease were to be sought for in the physical world. When the

1   1

growing knowledge of the functions of the nervous system began to disclose the connexion between mind and brain it seemed that in the sphere of mental disorders also physical causation might be established and physical remedies found. The materialistic tendencies of science in the eighteenth and nineteenth centuries led to an accentuation of this hope, and the tradition thus established, in which all consideration of the mind and its processes was eschewed in medical teaching, has been continued into our own time.

Nevertheless, the great clinical observers of those days did not fail to note the mental accompaniments of the bodily diseases which they treated with so much skill and sagacity, nor were they blind to the disorders of bodily functions which are associated with emotional stress or mental conflict. They paid much attention to the mental dispositions and physical characteristics of their patients, and endeavoured to confirm the correlation of particular diseases with particular " temperaments," which had been a tradition in medicine since the days of Hippocrates.   One of the temperaments they described was called the nervous or neurotic temperament, because those who had it were especially prone to suffer from nervous and mental disorders.

With the rise of neurology as a specialized department of medicine the need of a more precise knowledge of the part played by mental factors, both in the causation and in the treatment of morbid states, became more insistent, just because the connexion between the mind and the nervous system is more immediate and direct than that between the mind and the rest of the body.

It was frequently observed that nervous disorders, the symptoms of which seemed to be of a purely physical nature, were apparently produced by causes that were mainly, if not entirely, mental ; and sometimes it was seen that they were recovered from under circumstances which gave no support to the view that such disorders could have any physical foundation. But the physiological science of the time was deeply imbued with belief in the primacy of the physical side of the brain-mind relation, and it was not easy for men of those days to admit the possibility of any form of disease having its origin in the mind. We are, indeed, getting back to a somewhat similar belief at the present time, and the " behaviourist " school of psychology is busy translating the concepts of mental science into the language of physiology ; but, in the years between, fortunately for the Psychology of Medicine, we have been willing to work on the assumption that the mind is something real which is subject to its own laws and which may be the seat of processes that are of causal significance in relation to the incidence of mental and bodily disorders.

The acceptance of this assumption—quite irrespective of any metaphysical beliefs concerning the relations of body and mind—soon led to rapid advance in knowledge about the nature of those conditions which had come to be classed as " functional nervous disorders " ; and, incidentally, it also led to some new conceptions of mental structure and process which have left a permanent mark upon the science of psychology.

Two main lines of approach were open to the pioneers in this new field of inquiry : one was afforded by the age-long problem of Hysteria ; the other by the experimental research which became possible with the discovery of Hypnotism.   It seemed at first as if these two routes were separate and independent pathways to knowledge, but with fuller investigation it became clear that they were but different sides of the same road.   The early stages of this adventure were productive of much heat and controversy between the rival factions that took part in it, and with the fuller knowledge we now have it seems difficult to account for the animosities engendered by what ought to have been a dispassionate search for truth ; but in the light of more recent happenings in the same field the records of those days are peculiarly interesting and instructive, and they should serve as a warning to us at the present time to keep a watch on our feelings and our prejudices, and not allow them to influence our judgments in a sphere where they should have no place.

The later phases of the movement thus begun are outlined in the following pages, and the brief account there given circles round the names of two great men, both pioneers—Pierre Janet and Sigmund Freud.   The teachings of the former were at first received with doubt and suspicion ; those of the latter with vituperation and indignant denial of their truth.   There are special reasons why Freud's work should have brought upon him so much contumely and abuse ; but, even apart from these, the innate conservatism of the scientific world is perhaps sufficient to account for the widespread opposition which his revolutionary doctrines encountered.   It has been said that when Harvey discovered the circulation of the blood not one man in England who was at that time over forty years of age ever accepted the truth of this discovery.

The plan of this book is perhaps sufficiently indicated in the table of contents. The theory of " dissociation," elaborated by Professor Janet in connexion with his researches on hysteria and hypnotism is first considered. A short account of the main features of the hypnotic state and of hysteria as it was described by the older writers is followed by a brief consideration of the theory of dissociation and of the difficulty of applying it as an explanatory principle to all the observed phenomena. The theory of " repression," formulated by Professor Freud, is then taken up ; and the remainder of the book is devoted to an examination of the results which followed the utilization of this principle in the investigation of neurotic states. This necessitates an examination of the psycho-analytic conception of the " unconscious " and of the mechanisms of dream, and also some reference to psycho-analysis as a method of psychological investigation, as a body of doctrine, and as a therapeutic instrument. A summary description of the neuroses, founded upon the classification adopted by the psycho-analysts, is followed by an exposition of the principles underlying the various psychotherapeutic methods that have been employed in their treatment, and by some indication of the ground on which any mental hygiene directed towards the prevention of neurotic disorders should be based. In conclusion it is suggested that the opinions arrived at by different workers should be judged by different standards according as they are intent upon the attainment of scientific truth or upon finding the most practically useful way of dealing with those who suffer from neurotic disorders ; and that, even if no finality is to be expected in the opinions arrived at so far, there can be little doubt that psychology has been enriched and our outlook on human nature extended by the labours of those who have devoted their lives to a study of the Psychology of Medicine.

CHAPTER II

DISSOCIATION

(a) HYPNOSIS

THE psychological investigation of abnormal mental states may be said to have begun when Mesmer induced the scientific world to examine the phenomena of Animal Magnetism. Previous to this time, although unusual or disordered states of mind had often been observed and described, a psychology which was solely dependent on introspection could make little progress in elucidating their nature ; for the peculiarities of mental process which they displayed seemed to have little in common with anything the psychologist could discover in his own mind. Moreover, most of these states were met with only occasionally, they occurred only spontaneously, and they were often of short duration, so that any investigation undertaken was brought to an abrupt end with the termination of the abnormal condition. But when a means of inducing " magnetic trance " was discovered, an abnormal state, well deserving examination, could be brought about at will, and the first requisite of the experimental method —ability to repeat the experiment—was secured. It may be said that all our knowledge of the psychology of the abnormal can be traced to its beginnings in the study of artificially induced trance states.

But psychology, at this time, had not yet become emancipated from the trammels of metaphysical speculation, and the phenomena which Mesmer and his disciples ascribed to the virtues of the magnetic fluid received but scant attention from those whom training and interest should have, in some measure, fitted for the task of investigation.   The prejudice of the medical and scientific world of those days, assisted by the extravagance of the claims put forward by the Mesmerists themselves, succeeded in consigning to oblivion for many years this most important discovery.

During the whole of the Mesmeric period the methods of inducing the trance state were based upon Mesmer's doctrines.   The operator gazed fixedly at the patient because he believed that the eye was one of the principal outlets for the magnetic fluid.   He made passes over the patient's body because he believed that under the direction of the will the life-giving emanation oozed from his finger-tips.   All the resulting phenomena, inexplicable at that time by any of the known laws of nature, were ascribed to the mysterious new force which Mesmer thought he had discovered.

In 1843, James Braid, a Manchester surgeon, set himself to investigate the alleged facts of Mesmerism. He was soon convinced that at least one of the phenomena he observed was genuine.   He found that the mesmerized person was really incapable of opening his eyes.   Braid sought a physiological explanation of this, and he came to the conclusion that it resulted from the fatigue of the neuro-muscular mechanism brought into play in fixed gazing.   He found that fatigue of this kind is most readily produced when the object gazed at is sufficiently close to the eyes to cause a convergent squint, and that he could induce by this method a physical and mental state which appeared to be indistinguishable from the Mesmeric trance. To the state so induced he gave the name " Hypnotism, or nervous sleep."

Although Braid was at first inclined to explain his results as being due entirely to physiological fatigue, he soon discovered that the psychological side of his process had to be taken into consideration. In the further course of his studies he became more and more convinced of the importance of psychological factors in the hypnotizing process, and his later writings show that he ultimately regarded them as the only essential ones. He held the modern view that suggestion is the principal agent in the production of the hypnotic state and of all its associated phenomena. Braid's work was, however, soon forgotten, and it was not until Liébeault rediscovered the power of suggestion that the period of modern hypnotism can be said to have begun. The work of Liébeault might have shared a fate similar to that of Braid, had it not been his good fortune to have attracted the interest of Bernheim, a professor at Nancy, who championed his cause and spread his teaching throughout the world. With the rise of the Nancy school the belief that hypnosis can be induced by suggestion became widely accepted, and although the old physical or physiological hypothesis found some favour for a time, the methods everywhere employed by hypnotists at the present day are practically the same as those used by Liébeault and Bernheim.

The suggestion of sleep at the very beginning of the hypnotizing process is the distinguishing feature of the Nancy method, and almost all modern records of hypnotic phenomena describe what is observed when hypnosis is induced in this way. The reiterated suggestions of sleep tend to induce a feeling of drowsiness which is displayed even in the lighter stages of hypnosis, whilst in the deeper stages the resemblance to profound slumber is sometimes very pronounced. But besides the suggestions of sleep certain aids to suggestion are usually found to be of importance, such as a preliminary fixing of the gaze, repose of mind and body, and freedom from distracting disturbances of any kind. In very susceptible subjects these are relatively unimportant, but in most cases they are essential to success.

The hypnotic states brought about by these measures vary greatly in different people. In almost every instance, however, if any degree of hypnosis has been induced, the patient remains passive if he is left undisturbed. He shows no inclination to move or to speak, although he is quite capable of doing so. This passivity is almost as great in the light stages of hypnosis as in the deep stages, when the Nancy method is used, and it cannot, as a rule, be regarded as giving any indication of the depth of the hypnotic state induced. This can be ascertained only by noting how the subject responds to further suggestions.

Many attempts have been made to classify the stages or degrees of hypnosis, and all these attempts are based on the variations in susceptibility to suggestion which are observed in different persons, or in the same person at different times. Almost all the classifications thus made are more or less arbitrary, and they have little value either for descriptive purposes or as a guide in practical hypnotic work. But the transition from the ordinary waking state to profound hypnosis is so gradual that it is necessary to fix upon certain phenomena which may be taken as landmarks in surveying the whole field. It is important in the first place to decide at what point in the transition the hypnotic state may be regarded as definitely beginning ; and it is important also to take as another landmark the point at which the events of hypnosis cease to be remembered when waking life is resumed.

In practice it has come to be considered a useful rule to regard inability to open the eyes, when this inability is suggested, as indicating the definite onset of hypnosis. If this suggestion is effective other suggestions of a similar kind may be tried. It may be found possible to prevent closing the eyes, opening the mouth, swallowing, and other movements of a similar kind. If an attempt is made to inhibit movements such as walking or writing, the suggestions may or may not be effective. If they are effective it is generally held that the subject is in a deeper stage than that in which only movements such as opening the eyes can be inhibited. Further suggestions, which may be responded to in the deeper states, may then be tried, such as loss of cutaneous sensation, loss of memory of particular facts, illusions, hallucinations, delusions, and amnesia on awaking of all that has taken place during hypnosis. The kind of suggestion that will be effective in any particular case is supposed to depend on the depth of the hypnosis, but it must be remembered that the depth of the hypnosis is judged in the main by the kind of suggestions that are effective.

Both Liébeault and Bernheim divided hypnotic states into two great groups, namely, light sleep states, the events of which are remembered on awaking, and deep sleep states, the events of which are not remembered on awaking. It is recognized by almost all writers that the most important dividing line in any classification is where forgetfulness of the events of hypnosis begins to appear. When post-hypnotic amnesia is complete it is customary to describe the degree of hypnosis by the term somnambulism.

The most common conditions of memory in connexion with the transitions from waking to hypnosis and from hypnosis to waking again may be told in a few words ; but some of the peculiarities that may be observed are difficult to describe and still more difficult to interpret. If a person in any stage or degree of hypnosis be interrogated, he will invariably be found to have knowledge of his past life as complete, at least, as he has in the waking state. In the deeper stages it may be found that memory of his past life is more complete and more extensive than during waking life. If he is awakened and questioned as to his experiences during hypnosis his recollection of what has transpired may be clear or hazy, or altogether absent. But whatever defects of recollection of the events of hypnosis he may exhibit in the post-hypnotic waking state, the memory of these events will immediately be restored to him when he is again hypnotized. In this respect, at least, the memory in hypnosis is more extensive than in the waking state. A hypnotic somnambule can remember during hypnosis both the events of his normal life and the events of previous hypnoses ; in his waking state he can remember only the events of his previous waking states—his normal life.

Of all the differences between the state of the mind in hypnosis and in ordinary waking life none is so distinctive as that which is found in regard to the action of suggestion. In the waking state, suggestion under certain conditions may have noteworthy effects on belief and conduct ; but these are far surpassed by those that are obtained in the hypnotic state. Not only is response to suggestion during hypnosis evoked more easily and more certainly than in the waking state, but suggestibility is manifested in regard to a much wider range of phenomena, and reveals some unsuspected powers in the psycho-physical organism. In response to suggestion voluntary muscular movements may be augmented, or diminished to the extent of complete paralysis ; the normal periodicity of involuntary muscle functioning may be modified ; secretions may be induced, increased, diminished or arrested ; sensory acuteness may be sharpened, or blunted to the point of complete anæsthesia and analgesia ; hallucinations of the senses, obsessions and delusions may sometimes be brought about.

An important aspect of the results of suggestion presents itself in connexion with the post-hypnotic amnesia of somnambules. It is a noteworthy fact that any or all of the events of hypnotic somnambulism may be remembered on awaking if the operator gives a suggestion to that effect. The amnesia following the most profound hypnosis may be entirely avoided by a simple suggestion that everything that happens during the trance shall be remembered. It has been questioned, therefore, whether the loss of recollection which so constantly follows deep hypnosis may not always be due to conscious or unconscious suggestion by the hypnotist, or to self-suggestion based on the popular belief that hypnosis necessarily entails unconsciousness.

In a great many instances post-hypnotic amnesia is undoubtedly a consequence of deliberate suggestions of forgetfulness given by the operator. Such suggestions are indeed the readiest means of hastening the onset of somnambulism. On the other hand, hypnosis is often followed by amnesia when no suggestion of forgetfulness has been given. It is practically impossible, however, to eliminate self-suggestion, and to those who believe that there is nothing in hypnotism but suggestion, this will always appear to be the true explanation of post-hypnotic amnesia.

We may, however, miss the significance of much that is of importance if we press the principle of suggestion too far in the interpretation of hypnotic phenomena ; and fertile though this principle has been in bringing order out of confusion, its indiscriminate application sometimes tends to complicate what is otherwise relatively simple, rather than to afford any useful solution of our difficulties. Instead of reiterating the dictum of Bernheim that there is nothing in hypnotism but suggestion, let us recognize that hypnosis is a psychologically distinct state or phase of consciousness, characterized by certain definite peculiarities. This state comprises various grades, or degrees of completeness, in all of which increased suggestibility is found, and in some of which the phase of consciousness is of such a nature that spontaneous recollection of what happens during hypnosis is impossible when normal life is resumed.

It is the occurrence of post-hypnotic amnesia that gives the chief interest to those results of suggestion during hypnosis which are included under the misleading designation of post-hypnotic suggestion. A post-hypnotic suggestion is not a suggestion given after hypnosis is terminated, but a suggestion given during hypnosis and fulfilled at a later time, either in the waking state or in a subsequent hypnosis. Amnesia of the suggestion is not essential, but when amnesia does occur it renders the success of the experiment more striking, and it raises some psychological problems of considerable importance. The fulfilment of suggestions of this kind throws some light on the apparent discontinuity of mental process which leads up to many compulsive and instinctive actions, and the known source of the ideas which determine post-hypnotic actions may prepare us for the knowledge that many of the activities of ordinary life are likewise determined by ideas existing below the normal threshold of consciousness.

There are two points of special interest connected with the performance of post-hypnotic acts. The first relates to the mental state of the subject when a post-hypnotic suggestion is being fulfilled ; and the second has reference to the memory of this event in subsequent waking life. It is often noticed that a person engaged in the performance of a post-hypnotic act does not seem to be his normal self and that he may afterwards forget more or less completely what he has done. Investigation seems to show that post-hypnotic acts may be performed in a variety of different states. These states may show gradation between what is to all appearance ordinary waking, and a condition which is indistinguishable from hypnosis. The abnormality of many of these states may be shown in various ways. In some cases it is sufficiently indicated by the appearance of the subject. More conclusive, however, is the discovery that during the performance of post-hypnotic acts there may be increased suggestibility. Still further it is found that during this abnormal state there may be recollection of the events of previous hypnoses. Moreover, acts performed in the post-hypnotic state may be forgotten immediately afterwards.

All these facts point to the probability that the abnormal state in which post-hypnotic suggestions are fulfilled is itself a hypnotic state. But although there is obviously some relation between abnormal states of this kind and true hypnosis, it cannot be overlooked that in most instances there is some difference. The most commonly observed difference is that whilst all the events of hypnosis are forgotten on waking, the amnesia following these states is confined to the post-hypnotic act alone.

The simultaneous occurrence of activities apparently guided by two separate intelligences which is exhibited in post-hypnotic experiments points to the conclusion that we have in these cases a transient manifestation of a sort of doubling of consciousness which we meet with in more fully developed forms in certain types of multiple personality. The idea conveyed in a post-hypnotic suggestion becomes subliminal when waking life is resumed, and the fulfilment of the suggestion is accompanied by a subliminal invasion of the waking consciousness to such extent only as is necessary for the adequate performance of the suggested act. The extent to which the waking consciousness is thereby displaced depends on the extent to which the activities of the whole organism are involved in the fulfilment of the suggestion. If only a limb movement is in question there may be no apparent departure from the normal state, and if the movement is noticed by the subject he may remember having made it. But if the fulfilment of the suggestion necessitates a complicated series of movements demanding attention to diverse bodily activities, or if a post-hypnotic hallucination has been produced, the whole waking consciousness may become displaced while the hypnotic consciousness comes to the fore.

When we take into consideration the facts of post-hypnotic amnesia and the acquisition by the hypnotic consciousness of many memories which never become a possession of the waking self, we are almost justified in thinking of the hypnotic personality as something distinct and separate from the waking personality. But in so far as personality consists of an organized system of mental dispositions we can find little difference between the waking and the hypnotized person. If suggestion is avoided a person in hypnosis will be found to possess all the knowledge that he has in ordinary life ; he will show the same likes and dislikes, and the same purposes and ends. But if he is not questioned he remains passive. He is not asleep, yet he is not awake. He is capable of mental activity, but he scarcely exhibits any. The stream of consciousness seems to stagnate. The flow of ideas determined by interest and association in waking life now hardly seems to occur. What mental activity there is seems to be determined wholly from without. In waking life the modification of conscious states by extraneous conditions depends on the interest which attaches to the determining factors, but the flow of thought is, to a large extent, self-sustaining. In the hypnotic state interest seems restricted to the person who has induced the hypnosis, and in the absence of determination from this source mental

2

activity seems as a rule to be extremely restricted. The striving aspect of mental life seems to be absent, unless, indeed, it exists as a desire or inclination to fulfil the suggestions of the hypnotist.

This description is more applicable to the state of mind in deep hypnosis induced for the first time than to that which obtains after the subject has been hypnotized many times, and has undergone " training " through experimentation, or through having been frequently conversed with in the hypnotic state and treated as if he were his ordinary waking self. In almost every instance when this is done the state of mind during hypnosis approximates much more nearly to that which we regard as characteristic of waking life ; the consciousness of the hypnotized person once more becomes a stream that flows. Trains of thought determined from within arise, and some degree of spontaneous behaviour—spontaneous speech or other movements— may appear ; there is, as it were, a new organization of personality at the hypnotic level of consciousness. The self thus formed is not in all respects identical with the waking self, and, in some rare cases, may show very different characteristics. Always, however, the hypnotic self knows what is known by the waking self, and, in addition, it knows what it has learnt during its own phases of activity. Brought into being by a narrowing of the field of consciousness it is soon enabled to envisage in its outlook the whole of the normal field, and even much that lies beyond its boundaries. It includes within its structure all the mental dispositions whose functional activity manifests in waking consciousness, but it also includes dispositions which only subconsciously affect the waking life.

In the great majority of instances the modifications of personality revealed in the hypnotic state are very slight. The hypnotic personality is not different from the waking personality except in that it has at its command recollections of experiences which the waking personality cannot voluntarily recall, and in the relative absence or abeyance of the striving aspect of mental life. In a small number of cases, however, the personality arising or appearing in the hypnotic state differs so much from that of the waking, and presumably normal, self, that such cases must be regarded as genuine examples of double or multiple personality. The study of these conditions belongs to the topic of Hysteria which must next be considered.

(b) HYSTERIA

The mental and physical abnormalities which are included under the term hysteria have been known in some measure from the earliest times, but it is only within the last forty years that any reasonable interpretation of them has been possible. After a long period during which knowledge of hysteria was merely descriptive, the great clinical observers of the nineteenth century devoted themselves to classification of the innumerable disabilities of hysterical patients, and so brought some order into what had been, for centuries, a mere collection of unconnected symptoms. But so diverse were the defects and peculiarities that had been observed and described, so little did they seem to be related one to another, so various and inconstant were the conditions which led to their occurrence, that it was hard to find any factor which would help to bind together these seemingly unrelated phenomena.

It is not necessary to describe in detail the various symptoms of hysteria, but it is important for us to know in a general way the kinds of defect which occur, and to bear in mind the peculiarities which stamp these defects as hysterical affections.   Countless in number, inexhaustible in kind, there are yet certain features which are common to all hysterical symptoms, and it is the possession of these common features that justifies us in classifying under the term hysteria so many defects which at first sight appear to be totally unrelated one to another.

In the description of hysteria by the great clinicians of former years it was a common practice to divide the symptoms into two groups.   In one group were placed the paroxysmal attacks or " fits " to which the hysteric is liable.   In the other group were included the many disabilities that may be observed in the absence of any definite paroxysm, or as more or less permanent symptoms in the intervals between the attacks.   The most common paroxysmal manifestation is the ordinary hysterical fit or convulsion.   This varies greatly in severity.   In the slighter attacks there may be no appearance of loss of consciousness, but in others the patient may appear to lose touch with his surroundings, and on recovery may have no recollection of the incidents of the attack.

The convulsion or fit, however, occupies but a small part of the field of hysterical affections.   Persisting bodily and mental symptoms of the most varied kind occupy the greater part.   There is no function of the body that may not be implicated, and the disabilities so produced sometimes simulate very closely those due to grave organic disease.   For our present purpose it will suffice to refer to one or two of the most common forms of sensory and motor defect, and we may omit any reference to the purely mental disorders that may arise.

Anæsthesia was regarded by Charcot as the great stigma of hysteria, and although it is not now believed to have the diagnostic importance formerly ascribed to it, it is one of the most common features of the disorder and the one best suited for study as a type of hysterical disability. Every region of the body and every form of sensibility may be affected. When anæsthesia is not widespread the localization of the affected areas is often very characteristic. These areas do not correspond to parts supplied by any particular nerve or nerves. They do not conform to any anatomical division of the body but rather to popular conceptions or the rough practical divisions of ordinary speech. Thus, for example, the hand is commonly regarded as a portion of the body clearly marked off from the rest of the arm, and a hysteric may get anæsthesia which terminates abruptly at the wrist. And so with regard to the foot, the arm, the leg, and other parts of the body, the distribution of hysterical anæsthesia is not such as can be accounted for by organic lesion. The anæsthetic areas may be confined to isolated patches of various shapes which have always this peculiarity, that they correspond to some idea in the patient's mind rather than to any anatomical fact.

The anæsthesia may be profound and persistent, yet there is no trophic disturbance of the skin, no sores form, nor are the affected parts specially liable to injury as happens in organic anæsthesia. Accompanying the anæsthesia of hysteria we find a strange indifference to its presence. The patient is often unaware of any defect until it is revealed in the process of examination. The sufferer from organic anæsthesia is often acutely conscious of his loss of sensibility, but the hysteric is indifferent to a similar loss even when its existence is demonstrated to him by the physician.

Although loss of sensibility appears to be profound, yet it may be shown that some sort of awareness of sensory stimulation is present. Sensation is not wholly lost as it is in organic anæsthesia. Although the patient has no supraliminal perception of impressions, such as pin pricks, on the anæsthetic area, yet it can be shown by various devices that perception is still present in some subliminal form. The subliminal perceptions of the hysteric may give rise to thoughts of which the patient is aware. Thoughts that seem to arise spontaneously can be shown to be due to stimulations of which there is no supraliminal perception. Thus, for example, if the anæsthetic arm be screened from the patient's vision and pricked a number of times, the patient on being asked to mention the first number that occurs to him may very likely give the number corresponding to the number of pricks. Subliminal perception is also revealed by the movements of adaptation which take place when some common object is put into the anæsthetic hand. A pencil or a pair of scissors, for example, will be held in a way appropriate to its use—a result which could not occur if there were not some recognition of the object.

Hysterical anæsthesia is very commonly accompanied by a loss or diminution of movement in the affected part. This paralysis may sometimes closely resemble that due to organic disease, but as a rule there are so many points of difference that diagnosis is not difficult.

In the realm of sensation hysterical disorders may take the form of hyperæsthesia rather than anæsthesia, and in regard to movement it may lead to excess rather than diminution of muscular activity. Various forms of spasmodic contraction—choreic movements, tics, and tremors—may occur ; or there may be a continuous steady contracture of a group of muscles which keep a limb in one position for an indefinite time.

The peculiarities, thus briefly indicated, which pertain to anæsthesia and paralysis in hysteria, are but examples of the difficulties which beset the early workers when they tried to bring this disorder into line with their knowledge of other states. Charcot, applying the clinical methods of which he had made so masterly a use in his investigations of other diseases of the nervous system, sought in the physiological domain for general laws that might be applicable to the whole range of hysterical disabilities. But although it is to Charcot's initiative that we owe the widespread interest in hysteria which obtains at the present time, it is now generally admitted that his too close adherence to ordinary clinical methods led him into many errors. It is to Bernheim that we owe the beginnings of those psychological interpretations which dominate all the best work on hysteria at the present day.

The modern developments of the psychological conceptions put forward in explanation of hysterical phenomena may be said to have had their starting-point in the controversy which took place between the Paris and the Nancy schools concerning the nature of hypnotism and its relation to hysteria. The undoubtedly close resemblance between hysterical and hypnotic phenomena was admitted by both sides. But Charcot and his pupils had studied hypnotism in hysterical persons only, while Bernheim and his colleagues declared that they had induced hypnosis in about 90 per cent. of ordinary hospital patients. It was admitted by both sides that hysterical phenomena can be produced by suggestion and that hysterical patients are very suggestible. Thus two extreme views of the relation of hysteria to hypnosis came to be held. On the one hand it was taught that all hysterical symptoms are due to suggestion, and on the other that all suggestion is due to hysteria.

At the present time there are two outstanding conceptions of hysteria which hold the attention of students of abnormal psychology. One has been elaborated by Professor Pierre Janet of Paris, and the other by Professor Sigmund Freud of Vienna. Freud's work, so far at least as publication of his results is concerned, is the later of the two, and his doctrines differ profoundly from those of Janet. But both doctrines have, at least, this in common, that they try to explain hysteria entirely in psychological terms. And since the explanation of hysteria and other neuroses in psychological terms forms the main subject matter of the Psychology of Medicine it is necessary to examine in some detail the views of these two writers.

All Janet's studies of hysteria centre in the problem of the trance state which he terms *somnambulism*. The most common or best known form of somnambulism is the sleep-walking such as is depicted by Shakespeare in the fifth act of Macbeth. In this scene Lady Macbeth appears carrying a lighted taper. Her eyes are open, but, as the gentlewoman says, " their sense is shut." She rubs her hands and speaks. She is evidently living again through the scene of the murder, and giving voice to the thoughts that accompanied it. Similar though less tragic episodes are often enacted during sleep by ordinary people, especially children, and it is indeed an everyday experience to meet men or women who say they have walked in their sleep at some period of their lives.

Conduct in some ways similar to that of the sleep-walker is often observed in hysteria, and Janet considers the fit of somnambulism which appears spontaneously in hystericals to be the most typical, the most characteristic, symptom of this disorder. It occurs in many forms and degrees which, though differing widely in appearance, are nevertheless all constructed on the same model. The simplest and most easily understood form is that which Janet calls *monoideic*. One of the cases recorded by him may serve as an illustration. A young girl, twenty years old, nursed her dying mother. The poor woman, who had reached the last stage of consumption, lived alone with her daughter in a poor garret. Death came slowly with suffocation, blood-vomiting, and all its frightful procession of symptoms. The girl struggled hopelessly against the impossible. She watched her mother during sixty nights, working at her sewing machine to earn a few pennies necessary to sustain their lives. After the mother's death she tried to revive the corpse, to call the breath back again ; then, as she put the limbs upright the body fell to the floor, and it took infinite exertion to lift it again into the bed. Some time after the funeral the young girl began to fall into somnambulic attacks in which she acted again all the events that took place at her mother's death, without forgetting the least detail.

One of the characteristics of these somnambulisms is

that they repeat themselves indefinitely. Not only are the different attacks always alike, repeating the same movements, expressions and words, but in the course of the same attack the same scene may be repeated exactly in the same way many times.

An attack of somnambulism may begin suddenly or slowly. When the onset is sudden there is a sort of faint and a seeming loss of consciousness. When it is slow there is a gradual abasement of mental activity. When the state has been entered its most important characteristics are the perfection and intensity of the development of the dream, the marvellous plasticity of the expressions and attitudes, the apparent vividness of the hallucinations, the fluency of elocution and eloquence of diction, and the precision and quickness of the movements. All these peculiarities are exhibited in a degree that is quite beyond the powers of the patient in the waking state.

The development of the somnambulic delirium is perfectly regular, and the various episodes are exactly repeated every time it occurs. During the attack the senses are shut to all impressions not connected with the dream, the patient perceives nothing except the idea he is possessed of, and he remembers nothing except that one idea. With the end of the somnambulism comes a return of all sensations, the lost memories of waking life are restored and the events of the somnambulism are forgotten. Thus there is during the crisis a huge unfolding of all the phenomena connected with a certain delirium, and an absence of every sensation and every memory not connected with the delirium. After the crisis there is a return of consciousness, of sensations, and of normal memory, and entire forgetfulness of all that is connected with the somnambulism. This loss of memory bears not only on the period of the somnambulism, on the scene of the delirium ; it bears also on the event that has given birth to that delirium, on all the facts that are connected with it, on the feelings that are related to it. Thus the young girl referred to forgot, during her waking state, all the events connected with her mother's illness and death. She was callous and insensitive and her filial love, the feeling of affection she had felt for her mother, seemed to have quite vanished. Monoideic somnambulism is followed by an amnesia which bears not only on the somnambulism itself, but also on all the facts and memories related to it.

The psychological explanation of somnambulism given by Janet is well known. Somnambulism is due, he says, to a *dissociation* of consciousness. An idea or partial system of thoughts, such as the memories connected with a mother's death, becomes separated from the great body of ideas and memories which constitute the personal consciousness. The dissociated system of thoughts becomes independent and develops on its own account. Emancipated from the control of the infinitely wider system of thoughts with which normally it is connected, and to whose laws it is subject, it tends to develop to excess, and consciousness appears no longer to control it. In the intervals between the somnambulic attacks the ideas thus dissociated remain subconscious, but when, in any way, an effective appeal to them is made, they come to the surface, as it were, displace the great mass of ideas forming the personal consciousness, and dominate the organism for so long as the somnambulism lasts.

Taking as a starting-point the monoideic type of

somnambulism and his psychological interpretation of its mechanism, Janet applies the conception of dissociation as an explanatory principle to every kind of hysterical symptom. Mental dissociations may be ranged in a series, at one end of which we find functional anæsthesia of limited extent, tics or paralyses affecting particular movements, amnesia of isolated events or bearing upon short periods of time ; at the other end are those profound dissociations which are known as double or multiple personalities.

For not all somnambulisms are monoideic. There is another group which Janet calls *polyideic*, in which several ideas or emotional experiences are dissociated from the personal consciousness, and may be enacted one after another during the somnambulism. Although, at first sight, these dissociated memories may appear to be unrelated to each other, it may be found that they have some underlying feeling or emotion in common, so that the various episodes reproduced in the somnambulism may all be recognized as variations of the same theme. During the acting out of the different scenes, the somnambulist, just as in the monoideic form, is almost entirely engrossed in his dream, and his senses are not sufficiently awake to bring him into touch with the real world. But there are some polyideic somnambulisms in which impressions from without do enter into and modify the dream. If ability to perceive and appreciate the nature of surrounding objects be retained, the regular development of the somnambulism may be interfered with and modified by the performance of actions determined by the actual situation. In other cases still further modifications may be introduced by association of ideas.

In most of these cases conduct consists mainly of actions appropriate to past events in the patient's history, and is not relevant to his actual circumstances during the somnambulism. When the dissociation is of such a nature as to permit a just appreciation of the surroundings during the secondary state, and ability to react in an appropriate manner, there is a tendency for the state to be prolonged, and to be filled up by a course of conduct in which are displayed the purpose and contingency which we regard as characteristic of waking life. Attacks of this kind usually take the forms of *fugues* or ambulatory automatisms.

Fugues are of not infrequent occurrence, and many of the cases of lost memory reported from time to time in the newspapers are of this character. These people have lost for the time being the memory of their real personality. Some system of thoughts which determines their wanderings has become dissociated from the personal consciousness. As is the tendency of all dissociated ideas this system of thoughts takes on independent functioning, and when it is working itself out in action the other systems of thoughts relating to the personality, to the former life and its responsibilities, become latent. The whole personality is no longer in control of conduct. When through some chance association, or through artificial means, the memory of the former existence is restored, the lately active system of thoughts becomes latent again and the events associated with its recent activity are forgotten.

From fugues to one type of alternating double personalities is but a step. The well-known case of Ansel Bourne may be taken as an example of this type. Ansel Bourne suddenly forgot who he was, assumed a new name and for a fortnight wandered about from city to city. He then settled down as a small shop-keeper and continued for six weeks to live an uneventful life in his secondary state. During all this time he had no recollection of his former life. Then he woke up one morning in his proper personality and forgot all the events of his secondary state.

Several cases have been recorded in which there has been such reciprocal amnesia between the two states ; A does not know B, and B does not know A. The memory relations between the two states are in these cases different from those which subsist between the hypnotic state and the waking consciousness. On the other hand, there are many cases of double personality in which the secondary state has the same relation to the primary state as the hypnotic consciousness has to the waking consciousness. In these cases A does not know B, but B does know A—knows all A's thoughts, feelings, and actions, and knows them as belonging to A. Because of the concomitant awareness exhibited in these cases they may be referred to as belonging to " the co-conscious type " of double personality. Some modern examples of this type have been exhaustively studied and recorded in great detail, notably the Beauchamp case by Dr. Morton Prince, and the Doris Fischer case by Dr. Walter F. Prince.

An important characteristic of monoideic somnambulisms, and of all somnambulisms constructed on the same model, is that the attacks can be artificially reproduced. We have only to awaken in the mind of the subject, in a more or less precise manner, the idea whose development fills up the somnambulism, to cause the latter to reappear. The states thus artificially reproduced are not long in being a little modified. When once the experimenter has established relations with the dream consciousness of the subject, he may impart to it ideas which can develop without stopping the state. At first he can only be understood by the subject if he speaks of ideas related to the somnambulic dream, but he is soon himself a part of the dream, and is heard and understood if he speaks of anything whatever. "Thus," says Janet, "is formed in some subjects an artificial somnambulism which has been given the name of hypnotism."[1]

This account of what hypnotism is has never been accepted by followers of the Nancy School. It seems to be opposed to the experience of every practical hypnotist. Janet says that the hypnotic state is nothing but the reproduction of an hysterical somnambulism in an hysterical subject, and that in every one in whom the state can be induced examination will show a past history of hysterical disorders. They are, he says, "mostly hysterical patients, having already had somnambulism in some form or other, or for the remaining part hysterical patients having presented other accidents, but having the mental state characteristic of hysteria."[2] On the other hand, Bernheim and Liébeault, and those who have adopted their theories and methods, maintain that they can induce hypnosis, to a greater or less degree, in from 80 to 90 per cent. of ordinary people, in most of whom no history of any antecedent hysterical effection can be discovered.

It cannot be maintained that 80 or 90 per cent. of ordinary people are hysterical in any useful sense of the word, or that they have suffered from hysterical somnam-

[1] *The Major Symptoms of Hysteria*, p. 114.
[2] *Ibid*, pp. 114, 115.

bulisms. If they possess any of the qualifications desiderated by Janet for the occurrence of hypnosis, these must be found in their having, in his less committal phrase, " the mental state characteristic of hysteria." And it would indeed seem likely that there is some mental state or predisposition common to those who suffer from hysteria, and to those who can most readily be hypnotized.

The occurrence of both hysteria and hypnosis may be dependent on such predisposition, but this does not imply that hysteria and hypnosis are identical. We may suppose that some special capacity for dissociation is the one qualification necessary both for the occurrence of hysterical symptoms and for the induction of hypnosis. A person who can be hypnotized is a person who may, under appropriate circumstances, become an hysteric, but who need not already have suffered from any manifest hysterical disability. We should guard against Janet's implication that every dissociation is evidence of hysteria, for, as we shall see later, some amount of dissociation is common to all human beings. We should restrict the word hysterical to dissociations which arise spontaneously and result in defects or disabilities, and we should reserve the word hypnotic for those which are artificially produced.

(c) THE THEORY OF DISSOCIATION

Although the principle of dissociation is commonly accepted as applying equally to every phase and variety of hysterical affections, and to every stage or degree of hypnosis, it will be found that certain difficulties arise when we try to conceive the real nature of the dissociative mechanism if it is assumed to be the same in all of them. Looked at from the side of the waking consciousness the matter seems simple enough. When dissociation occurs, something that has been in consciousness becomes split off or dissociated from it. The immediate result of such a splitting off is an amnesia—a forgetfulness, an inability to recall certain thoughts or feelings or actions. It may be a loss of memory of a group of sensations or of movements, resulting in anæsthesia or paralysis, or it may be a forgetfulness of certain thoughts or events with all their associated feelings and activities.

That is what appears from the side of the waking consciousness ; it tells us nothing of what happens to the dissociated portions. But by various devices it can be shown that the dissociated thoughts are not non-existent, the dissociated sensations are not unfelt, the dissociated movements are not impossible of accomplishment. If a patient showing such amnesia be hypnotized, the forgotten events can be recalled, the lost sensations can be restored, the paralysed limb can be made to move. There is, however, plainly a division of consciousness, and from the side of the waking self there is no evidence of any commerce between the two parts. Amnesia is here the criterion of dissociation. But viewed from the side of the dissociated portion their relations to each other are not so clear. The dissociated ideas are, without doubt, cut off from the waking self, and Janet seems to imply that they are cut off from any possible self and are free to develop on their own account. But thoughts and feelings cannot be left floating about in the void, unclaimed by any thinker. We have no knowledge of any thoughts or feelings that are not the thoughts or feelings of some personal self. And we know

3

that in becoming dissociated the split-off portions do not necessarily lose their quality of consciousness. While the patient is awake and aware of some things, dissociated sensations or perceptions may provide evidence of a concurrent discriminative awareness of other things, as effective as that which characterizes the sensory or perceptive activity of the conscious waking self.

The problem of such concurrent awareness or co-consciousness greatly complicates the question of the nature of the dissociative mechanism in hysteria and hypnosis. So long as we are dealing with monoideic somnambulism, or with alternating personalities which show reciprocal amnesia and no co-consciousness, the conception of mental dissociation is relatively simple. The mind seems to be split into two parts, one of which exhibits conscious activity at one time, and the other at another time. Each is unable to draw upon the memories of the other, or to establish spontaneously any associative connexion with it. The psycho-neural dispositions, whose activity is manifested in each phase respectively, would seem to be totally dissevered from those pertaining to the other. A does not know B, and B does not know A, and the dissociation is shown in passing from A to B, as well as in passing from B to A.

In co-conscious states, such as ordinary hypnotic somnambulisms and co-conscious personalities, the dissociation shows itself in one direction only. The primary consciousness is cut off from all direct knowledge of the secondary state, but the secondary state has continuous and far-reaching knowledge of the primary state. There is an interesting experiment that may be tried with any trained somnambule—with any subject who can instantaneously be put into deep hypnosis by a prearranged signal and instantaneously awakened in the same way. Whilst he is in the normal waking state a conversation is opened on some topic which interests him. In the midst of the conversation the signal for hypnosis is given, and the conversation is proceeded with as if nothing had happened to interrupt it. It is immediately apparent that there is no break in the continuity of the subject's memory when he passes from the waking to the hypnotic state. He is quite aware of the topic of the conversation, and will continue to discuss it so long as the operator plies him with questions or asks for information. Or the conversation may be turned towards some other topic which may deal with any matter within the subject's knowledge. Throughout the whole conversation, if no attempt be made to impose suggestions upon him, he will show the range and limitations of his knowledge and interest ; he will express judgments from which his character may be gauged ; he will appear to be the same person in almost every way as he is in his normal waking life.

Yet there are some differences, almost always noticeable, which clearly indicate that the subject is not in his normal waking state. The most striking and constantly observed difference is the passivity, both bodily and mental, and the lack of spontaneity or initiative exhibited by the hypnotized person when he is not asked to speak or to act. He must be constantly stimulated by the questions and remarks of the hypnotist or the conversation lags. If the hypnotist ceases to ask questions or to make comments, the subject soon lapses into silence. In some cases occasional manifestations of spontaneity may be observed, but in my own experience I have found it to be an almost invariable rule that a hypnotized person does not speak and does not act unless he is directly or indirectly asked to do so.

When, at the end of such a conversation as is described above, the subject is awakened by a signal, he will, if questioned, continue the conversation from the point at which he dropped into the hypnotic state, and he will again give the same answers and express the same judgments as he did during the hypnotic phase, seemingly in complete ignorance of having already gone over the same ground. The discontinuity of mental process which we should expect to accompany dissociation is thus plainly manifested in one direction only. There is no discontinuity in passing from the waking to the hypnotic state, whilst there is abrupt discontinuity in passing from the latter to the normal state.

The mechanism of dissociation in hypnotic and other co-conscious states must, therefore, be of such a nature that whilst the secondary state is dissociated from the primary state, the primary state is not dissociated from the secondary state. The secondary state can bring into associative connexion all the mental dispositions which are at the service of the primary state.

Most writers would seem to imply that when the section of consciousness dissociated is small, such as a localized anæsthesia, it maintains an impersonal existence on its own account and does not belong to any self, but that when the dissociated portion is sufficiently large, when it contains within itself sufficient variety and amount of mental material, it thereupon develops into a secondary personality. But it is impossible to draw any hard and fast line between the two groups, and we must suppose that underlying all the dissociations which manifest co-consciousness there is always a permanent substratum of the real personality of which all secondary personalities are but modifications. Such a conception would apply to all hysterical and hypnotic states. When there is a limited hysterical anæsthesia the waking self gets no sensations from stimuli applied to the affected area, but, as we have seen, these sensations are somehow felt ; and if they are felt, they must be felt by some self. So that even here we may say that there is a self that has these sensations and a self that has them not.

Apart from the dissociations *en masse* which characterize somnambulisms and secondary personalities the same principle has been applied to explain the action of suggestion and the induction of hypnotic states. Professor McDougall has told,[1] in terms of brain structure and function, what he thinks takes place when hypnosis is induced and when suggestion is most effective. We conceive the structure of the mind as consisting of an enormous number of mental dispositions, the activity of any one of which is controlled or inhibited by its connexion with the others. The cerebral aspect of mental dispositions must be thought of as complex functional groups of nervous elements or neurones. The neurones of each group are so intimately connected with each other that every such group or disposition always functions as a unit, and the activity of any particular group is controlled or inhibited by the activity of other groups with which it is connected. In the waking state the whole cerebrum is kept in a state of sub-excitement by the stimuli which continuously fall upon all the sense organs, so that any disposition which is excited to dominant activity at any moment—any idea which is present to consciousness—is kept within due bounds by

[1] *Encyclopædia Britannica*, 11th Edit., Vol. XIV, p. 205.

the inhibitory action of all the other systems of dispositions. But when hypnosis is being induced the stimuli from the sense organs are cut off, and thought is arrested, as far as possible. The tide of nervous energy in the neurones subsides in consequence, and the resistance to the passage of impulses from one group to another increases, so that a state of relative dissociation of neurones throughout the cerebrum ensues, and sleep tends to come on. But the hypnotist by his words and manipulations has kept one system of ideas in activity, namely, those related to himself ; and the neural systems corresponding to these ideas form a pathway through which any disposition or group of neurones may be stirred into action. The disposition so stimulated now acts with unusual force, being dissociated from the rival dispositions which normally control or modify its excitement, and the " development to excess " of the idea, of which Janet speaks, becomes possible. To the uninhibited force of the ideas so roused the peculiar efficacy of suggestion is ascribed.

Though such a conception is well fitted to explain most of the facts of hypnotism and suggestion, its application becomes difficult when we try to utilize it in explaining the mental status of a trained hypnotic somnambule. Here we have what is practically a secondary hypnotic personality, and while dissociation *en masse* of the secondary from the primary state is most strikingly shown, evidence of relative dissociation of mental dispositions *within* the secondary state is hard to find.

Moreover, as we have seen, the continuity of memory in passing from the waking to the hypnotic state does not seem congruous with the notion that a disjunction of neurones is the correlate of the mental dissociation.

The difficulty of applying this conception of the mechanism of dissociation in every case, has led me to suggest, elsewhere,[1] that the dissociated status of co-conscious secondary personalities may be more easily understood if we regard them as being due to alterations of thresholds, rather than to disaggregation of psychoneural dispositions or interrelated groups of neurones.

In Janet's opinion the primary defect in hysteria is the lowering of nervous tension, the exhaustion of the higher functions of the brain, which is met with in all neuropathic disorders. When this diminution of tension brings about a general lowering of all the functions Janet says there results a morbid state which he has described under the name of Psychasthenia. But in hysteria, in consequence of some unknown hereditary peculiarities, the defect is localized on some particular function or functions. There is thus not so much a weakening of consciousness as a whole, but a retraction of the conscious field. Certain functions drop out of consciousness because the power of personal synthesis is at fault. There is a " lack of power, on the part of the feeble subject, to gather, to condense his psychological phenomena, and assimilate them to his personality."[2]

Janet recognizes that his description of hysteria leaves many problems unsolved. The most important of these is to account for the localization and nature of the defect in any particular case. Some stress or emotional shock

[1] *Proceedings Soc. Psych. Research*, Vol. XXVI, pp. 257, 285.
[2] *The Major Symptoms of Hysteria*, p. 311.

in a predisposed individual may produce a lowering of nervous tension, and a consequent retraction of the field of consciousness, but why does the resulting defect take the form of a paralysis of the arm in one case, and that of loss of speech, or loss of sight, or persistent refusal of food in another ?

Besides the difficulties of accounting for the localization of hysterical defects there are other difficulties in Janet's conception of hysteria which his hypotheses raise rather than solve. His doctrine of dissociation as the basis of hysterical phenomena has been accepted in a general way by all competent critics, but there is no such unanimity of opinion in regard to his explanation of the way in which dissociation is brought about. He ascribes the capacity of " personal synthesis " to the maintenance of a certain level of nervous tension in the cerebral tissues. When this level falls too low the unity of consciousness is broken, the personal synthesis becomes defective, and a subconsciousness is formed. But he takes as the type of personal synthesis that " personal perception " which consists in the assimilation to the personal consciousness of those sensory impressions through which we obtain knowledge of objects in the external world. By so doing he seems to emphasize unduly the purely cognitive aspect of consciousness and to neglect the part played by the emotions and the will. It is true that strong emotion is admitted to be a common precursor of hysterical affections, but its importance is ascribed to its tendency to bring about a lowering of nervous tension, probably consequent on the accompanying fatigue, rather than to its own efficacy as a psychic force. Dissociation is for Janet a curtailment of capacity, passively submitted to by an enfeebled consciousness—a catastrophe in which the emotions and the will take no active part.

It is the recognition of the part played by the conations or will of the patient in the production of hysterical symptoms that marks off at the very outset the conception of hysteria put forward by Freud from that of Janet. Instead of regarding dissociation as a merely mechanical splitting consequent on *misère psychologique*, a letting go of certain functions because the personality is too feeble to hold on to them, Freud puts in the first line, as a determining factor of dissociation, the mental conflict that ensues when incompatible wishes or desires arise in the mind. The splitting of consciousness is explained dynamically as being due to a conflict of opposing forces within the personality. How such a conflict arises, what it signifies, and what it may lead up to, can best be understood by tracing the history of those researches into the nature of hysteria which are associated with Freud's name.

CHAPTER III

REPRESSION

ALL the best work on hysteria has been based on the practical motive of desiring to relieve the sufferings and disabilities of those afflicted by this disorder. The work of the French schools, both in Nancy and in Paris, brought out very clearly the extreme suggestibility of hysterical patients, and it was soon discovered that any particular symptom could readily be made to disappear if a suggestion to that effect were given during hypnosis. But it was also found that when one symptom was removed very often another, apparently quite different one, took its place, and that the cure of severe hysteria by suggestion alone was therefore a very difficult matter.

Some years before the publication of Janet's first work a Viennese physician, Joseph Breuer, who had as a colleague Sigmund Freud, hit upon a novel plan of dealing with hysteria. In a patient whom they were treating by hypnotism they found that some of the symptoms were permanently relieved whenever certain forgotten episodes in her life were recalled during hypnosis and free expression given to the'emotions which were attached to them. These episodes were occurrences after which the symptoms had first appeared, and it was found that on all of these occasions the patient had had to repress some strong emotional excitement instead of giving vent to it by appropriate words and deeds. Some psychical shock or trauma was received and the accompanying emotions were repressed. Thus, for example, this patient suddenly became unable to drink, and as it was a very hot summer she suffered much from thirst. She would take a glass of water in her hand, but as soon as it touched her lips, she would push it away as if she were suffering from hydrophobia. In hypnosis, one day, she was talking of her English governess, whom she disliked, and finally told, with every sign of disgust, how she had come into the room of the governess and how that lady's little dog, which the patient abhorred, had drunk out of a glass. Out of respect for the conventions she had remained silent. Now, after giving energetic expression to her restrained anger, she asked for water and drank a large quantity without trouble. She awoke from hypnosis with the glass at her lips, and the symptom thereupon vanished permanently.

The patient herself described this new mode of treatment as the " talking cure," and jokingly referred to it as " chimney sweeping." Breuer and Freud called it the " cathartic method." The giving vent to the emotion they termed " abreaction."

These pathogenic memories, revealed in hypnosis, were unknown to the patient in the waking state. They were, as Janet would say, dissociated memories. But in hypnosis memory was widened and their recall was possible.

When Freud, some years later, took up again, by himself, the researches which he had begun in collaboration with Breuer, he very soon found that not all the patients whom he wanted to cure could be hypnotized. He was, therefore, faced with the problem of how he could recover, from the patient, memories which the patient himself had forgotten.   Here Freud recalled to mind what he had seen in Bernheim's hypnotic clinic at Nancy.   He had seen Bernheim bring back to the waking consciousness the events of deep hypnosis by persistently assuring the patient that he could and would remember.   Freud therefore applied the same method to his neurotic patients in the waking state. When he came to a point at which the patient could apparently remember no more he assured him that he could remember and that the correct memory would emerge at the moment when he pressed his hand on the patient's forehead.   True, the right thought did not always come at once, but he found that the recollections so induced led surely if slowly towards the forgotten memories which underlay the symptom.

But he found this " pressure method " to be very exhausting.   It was as if the memories were all there ready to come up, but were prevented from doing so by some force against which he had to struggle.   The presence of such a force was shown by the resistance of the patient, and this resistance had to be overcome before he could be cured.   Therefore, Freud thought, this force which now caused the resistance to the emergence of the forgotten memories must be the force which had originally caused the forgetting. Thus arose in Freud's mind his great conception of *repression* as the dynamic cause of dissociation and amnesia.

His next problem was to find the nature of the force

which had caused the repression and led to the forgetting.
On reviewing the cases he had treated in this way he
found that all the forgotten memories were of the sort
that one does not care to remember and prefers to
forget. They were memories of events or of thoughts
whose recurrence to the mind was painful, and he came
to the conclusion that repression is a defence reaction
of the mind against ideas that are unbearable. Moreover,
he found that in all those experiences which had acted
as mental shocks and had led to hysteria, some wish
had been aroused which was incompatible with the
moral or cultural standards of the patient. There had
been a short conflict in the mind, and the struggle was
brought to an end by the repression of the unbearable
wish. As an example we may take the case of a young
girl analysed by Freud about this time. When her
sister married, this girl developed a great attachment
to her new brother-in-law. She looked upon it as mere
family tenderness, but her love was greater than she
knew. While she and her mother were away from home,
the sister fell seriously ill, and they were hastily sent
for ; but before they arrived home the sister died.
While she stood by her sister's death-bed there flashed
through her mind the thought, " Now he is free and
can marry me." This thought, which for a moment
revealed to her the intensity of her love for her brother-
in-law, revolted her, and it was immediately repressed.
She forgot that such a thought had ever occurred to her,
but she fell ill with severe hysterical symptoms. During
her treatment by Freud this wish again became conscious
and its revival was accompanied by intense emotional
excitement. As a result she was cured of her
hysteria.

In such a case as this we find dissociation and amnesia following mental conflict due to the presence in consciousness of two incompatible wishes or desires. On the one hand was the desire of the conscious personality to be all that a devoted sister should be under the sorrowful circumstances of the moment. On the other side was the selfish craving of the unconscious love which she had for her sister's husband. To accept the wish thus suddenly revealed to her, to regard it as natural and not blameworthy, was to her sensitive mind intolerable ; and the realization that she had entertained this wish, even for a moment, aroused in her mind a conflict so great that to allow it to continue would have been equally unbearable. The weight of the whole of the rest of her personality was cast against the distasteful wish, with the result that the mind was split. Something too painful to be entertained, or even contemplated, was pushed out of consciousness and forgotten, and, as a consequence, the patient fell ill.

So far, we see a resemblance to what may have happened to Janet's patient who forgot the events of her mother's illness and death. Here, also, thoughts too painful to be borne may have been pushed out of consciousness. The mechanism of repression would account for the dissociation in the one case as in the other. In both patients something painful that had been in consciousness became split off from the conscious personality. But the subsequent history of the dissociated portions of the mind was different in the two cases. In Janet's patient the whole complex of painful thoughts and feelings became from time to time re-animated *en masse*, and, overpowering, as it were, the personal consciousness, displaced it and took control of the body during the somnambulisms. In Freud's patient the repressed wish gave no direct indications of its existence until Freud discovered it in the course of his analysis; but the patient had hysterical symptoms of another sort, namely, bodily pains and disabilities.

How, then, it may be asked, does the repression of an unbearable wish give rise to hysterical symptoms? Mental conflict and the forgetting of painful experiences are common enough, but they do not always lead to hysteria. It would seem that in neurotics the repression is not complete enough, and it does not wholly succeed in keeping the painful wishes out of consciousness. The repressed wish is not destroyed but still exists, in some unconscious region of the mind, as a wish seeking satisfaction and striving to get back into consciousness. The repressing forces, though not strong enough to keep it out of consciousness altogether, are yet strong enough to prevent it from returning in its true form. But it succeeds in getting into consciousness by becoming so distorted that its true nature is not recognized. The painful feeling or affect originally attached to the wish gets separated from it and becomes converted into the bodily manifestations which we know as symptoms of hysteria. To this process Freud has applied the term *conversion*, and the form of hysteria in which it occurs is now generally called Conversion Hysteria. For it does not always occur even when the repression fails to keep the distasteful wish out of consciousness altogether. The possibility of conversion seems to depend on some native peculiarity which is not always present; and when this capacity for conversion is absent, defence of the personality against the unbearable idea is effected by a *displacement* of the painful affect on to some other idea which is not in itself unbearable. In this way phobias and obsessions arise and the form of hysteria in which these are found is called Anxiety Hysteria.

The occurrence of a splitting of consciousness in hysteria is thus seen to be admitted by both Janet and Freud ; but on Janet's hypothesis the splitting is due to an inability of the self to assimilate certain ideas and feelings which ought to belong to it. On Freud's hypothesis the splitting is due, primarily, not to an inability but to an unwillingness of the personality to accept or acknowledge certain experiences as its own. Besides this difference in these two explanations of the origin of dissociation, there is, or may be, a further difference in respect of the mental material which becomes dissociated.   In hysterical paralysis of the arm, on Janet's hypothesis, the ideas and feelings related to the use of the arm have become dissociated from the personal consciousness. But, according to Freud, dissociation in such a case bears primarily on a totally different system of ideas.   It bears on some unbearable wish which, after being dissociated through conflict and repression, becomes converted into this particular physical disability. But the motor disability is itself a dissociation as Janet has shown, and it is a dissociation not directly due to conflict and repression. It is the result of the conversion of the painful wish into a physical symptom.

When a conscious wish is repressed it may be said that a dissociation occurs in so far as something that was in consciousness has become split off from it ; but when the repressed wish tries to become conscious

again and succeeds only by becoming converted into a
paralysis or an anæsthesia, a further dissociation occurs ;
for here again something that was in consciousness
becomes split off from it—namely, the systems of
ideas related to the sensations or movements affected.
Although, then, the repression of a painful wish implies
some degree of dissociation it seems clear that the
dissociations underlying the symptoms of conversion
hysteria are not directly due to repression but to the
process through which psychical pain becomes changed
into physical manifestations ; they are not due to
the repression but to the repressed material coming
back into consciousness in a distorted or disguised
form.

Setting out from his discovery of the psychical
trauma and the repression of an unbearable wish as the
origin of hysterical symptoms, Freud soon found that
it was not only one event in the patient's life that had
led to the symptom, but that many events of a similar
kind were implicated. These had to be brought back
to consciousness in the reverse order of their occurrence,
and only when the chain had been traced to its last link
was relief finally achieved. Indeed it was made evident
that only by the presence in the mind of earlier repressions did the later ones have any pathogenic significance.
In the end it was found that the unbearable wishes
underlying hysterical symptoms could in every instance
be traced back to childhood.

It was also found, with singular regularity, that
these repressed wishes belonged to the sexual life of
the patient ; and this held true not only of the wishes
of adult life and adolescence, but also of the infantile
wishes. Freud's doctrine of " infantile sexuality " is

4

that which above all others has aroused the most violent opposition and controversy, but some of this opposition may be avoided if we take the trouble to understand exactly what Freud means when he speaks of the sexual life of childhood.

INFANTILE SEXUALITY

Every child born into the world brings with him tendencies, inherited from his human and pre-human ancestors, which are incompatible with the ethical and cultural standards of civilized man. These tendencies are chiefly related to those great organic needs whose satisfaction in the animal world is not regulated or impeded by any moral or æsthetic considerations. The gratification of organic needs is accompanied by pleasure, and the tendency to seek pleasure and avoid pain is, according to one school of moral philosophy, the ultimate driving force behind the activities of every living creature. The pleasurable sensations to be derived from his own body are one of the first interests of the child, and his tendency to repeat such actions as give him pleasurable sensations has to be checked by those who are responsible for his upbringing, whenever these actions are regarded as offending against the canons of decency or propriety which have been adopted by the community into which he is born.

The child finds certain regions of his body, such as the mucous membrane of the mouth, the anus and the urino-genital tract, to be particularly sensitive and to afford a special quality of pleasure, although he may derive pleasure of a similar kind from other regions of the body, especially the skin. Freud calls these

areas " erotogenic zones " because he considers the
peculiar quality of the pleasure derived from these
areas to be analogous to, and genetically connected
with, the sexual pleasure of adult life.

Besides the pleasure derived from erotogenic zones,
other tendencies or impulses, which can sometimes be
easily detected in the sexual life of adults, are found to
be independent sources of pleasure in childhood.   These
impulses exist in contrasted pairs of which the chief are
looking or peeping, and showing off or exhibiting the
body—(observationism and exhibitionism), and the
pleasure in inflicting pain (sadism), with its passive
counterpart, the pleasure in suffering pain (masochism).
In childhood all these tendencies go their own way seeking
pleasure independently of one another and have nothing
to do with sex in the ordinary sense of being related
to reproduction ; but in the development of the normal
sexual life, while some of them are completely repressed,
the others converge as it were, and come under the
domination of the genital zone and are taken over into
the service of procreation.

At first sight there seem very good grounds for
objecting to Freud's inclusion of all these tendencies
and activities of childhood under the term infantile
sexuality. Perhaps his best justification for having
done so is found in the fact that when these tendencies
persist into adult life, as they sometimes do, they are
unhesitatingly recognized by every one as sexual perversions. The man who delights in the infliction of
pain on the object of his love is recognized as a sadist,
and the woman who is unsatisfied unless ·her lover
beats her is a masochist. No one questions the sexual
character of Peeping Tom's act when he transgressed

the order imposed upon the citizens of Coventry and peered through his shutters at Lady Godiva. Exhibitionism is seen in its crudest form in the cases, so common in our law courts, of men who are tried and punished for exposing themselves to children or young girls. Masturbation in adolescent or adult life is but the recrudescence of an infantile habit which even in childhood may be recognized as having sexual significance. Thus those tendencies and activities of childhood which Freud includes under infantile sexuality do indeed seem to have a close connexion with activities which in adult life we unhesitatingly regard as sexual. This fact has led Freud to describe the sexual life of the child as *polymorph pervers.* His sexual life consists of all those tendencies which in the adult we call sexual perversions.

The satisfaction of these tendencies is originally pleasurable to every normal child, but reprehensible when judged by the moral or æsthetic standards of the community ; and therefore reprehensible also to the child when he reaches a certain stage of development. The forces which lead to their repression exist within the child's own mind—the painful emotions of shame, loathing or disgust, which may or may not require the spark of social disapproval to arouse them.

Such is the nature of the tendencies which Freud discovered to be the material on which repression primarily bears. Every child passes through a phase in which these tendencies and desires are manifested. As he grows older their gratification, originally pleasurable, becomes accompanied by a sense of shame and guilt, and he half-consciously tries to get away from them and forget them. Ordinarily they are repressed and

forgotten and no longer manifest in the conscious life.
But they are not abolished or destroyed. They persist
somewhere in the mind and have profound effects on
future character and conduct. This is perhaps the
most original and the most startling contribution
which Psycho-Analysis has made to our knowledge of the
human mind.

DISPLACEMENT AND CONVERSION

Freud's hypotheses of displacement and conversion
are based upon a novel conception of the connexion
between the ideational content of mental process and
the accompanying affect or feeling tone. He regards
" affect " as a form of psychical energy which has all
the attributes of a quantity, so that it can be increased
or diminished or dissipated. Being but loosely attached
to the memory-traces of ideas, it may become displaced
from one idea to another. Normally it is worked off in
psycho-motor activities, such as those subserving the
bodily expression of the emotions, and if it is not
dissipated in action it accumulates and causes discomfort, dissatisfaction or displeasure. When it has a
free outlet its discharge brings relief, satisfaction or
pleasure.

The theory of repression is based upon this relation
between pleasure and the discharge of affect ; and
the effect of repression is to prevent the discharge of
the affect of any instinctive impulse that has been
aroused, and thus to prevent its being transformed into
bodily expression and felt as pleasure. For to the
developed or developing personality the pleasurable
satisfaction of primitive impulses which culture and
morality have rejected would be too painful to be borne,

and the sole function of repression is to keep from consciousness the knowledge of such impulses.

The inhibited impulse is kept from consciousness by a steadily exerted pressure from the direction of consciousness, and against this pressure the impulse seeking affective discharge maintains a counter-pressure. Its energy is dynamic and must find some outlet. Normally this is effected by a diversion of the energy into analogous forms of activity which are socially acceptable and in accord with the cultural and ethical standards of the individual. But when, for any reason, this sublimation of the primitive impulse does not take place or is inadequate, the repressing forces may be too weak to keep out of consciousness entirely the pent up energy of the impulse. The relatively weakened repression, although still strong enough to deny this impulse its natural outlet, is not able to prevent the abnormal or indirect outlets afforded by displacement and conversion. In both of these ways the discharge of affect is effected and some relief or gratification is secured, so that both mechanisms serve as a means of defence against ideas which in their undisguised form would be unbearable.

In the course of mental evolution, the original function of repression—the keeping out of consciousness ideas that are truly unbearable—would seem to have become extended, so that the same mechanism is made use of to protect the conscious personality from ideas that are merely distasteful or unpleasant. Many of the forgettings of everyday life which seem to be fortuitous and motiveless may be shown to be due to repression. Very commonly the things we forget are the things we do not want to remember. On the other hand we

know that we forget many things that we ardently
desire to remember. But in these cases also, repression
may often be shown to be the cause of the failure of
recollection. Here, however, repression is generally
indirect in its action. The memory that cannot be
recalled may, in itself, be not at all unpleasant, but
it will be found to have associations with other memories
which are surcharged with painful feeling. When
necessary these painful memories themselves may be
easily recalled. A painful event may have too much
significance in our lives for us ever to be able to forget
it, even if we would—for example, the death of some
one we love. Yet repression comes to our aid in avoiding
the needless revival of the painful memory by causing
us to forget indifferent ideas which by association
would tend to recall it. The continuous action of
repression, throughout the whole of life, in preserving
consciousness from painful memories that might be
aroused in this way, may be held to account for much
of our failure to recall our past experiences. Some
writers go so far as to suggest that all forgetting may
be due to repression.

In his investigation of hysteria Freud found that the
repressions of later life were always dependent upon
pre-existing repressions of a like nature, and in ultimate
analysis, upon those repressions of childhood which
arise as a defence against the primitive tendencies
grouped by him under the term Infantile Sexuality.
These tendencies and the pleasure derived from their
satisfaction are put away from consciousness, and
in the normal individual are never allowed to come
into consciousness again. In the repressions of childhood
the first splitting of the mind occurs and the split-

off tendencies are relegated to some region of psychic life which is not illuminated by consciousness ; and there they remain seeking satisfaction, and finding it as best they may, so long as life lasts. This region of the mind Freud calls The Unconscious.

CHAPTER IV

THE UNCONSCIOUS

WHETHER dissociation be due to *misère psychologique* or to mental conflict and repression or to displacement and conversion, it is common ground that when it occurs, something that has been in consciousness becomes split off from it and cannot be recalled by any normal mental process. In this it differs from those contents of the mind which, though not in consciousness at the moment, may readily become so. Each of us has a store of knowledge and acquisitions upon which we can draw, and many of the events of our past can be revived in consciousness, as memories, without difficulty. But when memories are dissociated they cannot be recalled either spontaneously or in response to promptings which normally would lead to recollection. So long as they are not in consciousness —in the field of consciousness at any moment—both the ideas that can be recalled and the ideas that cannot be recalled may be said, in everyday language, to be unconscious ; in psychology, however, it has become necessary to distinguish clearly between these two kinds of ideas and between two kinds of unconsciousness. For in psychology, as in everyday speech, the terms conscious and unconscious, consciousness and unconsciousness, are often used ambiguously.

To be conscious implies, or ought to imply, present awareness ; and consciousness should refer only to the " field of consciousness " at any moment. But very often consciousness is used as a collective concept to denote the totality of mental processes, and by the older psychologists it was commonly used as the anti-thesis of " matter," very much as we now use the word " mind." Even up to the present time some people think that consciousness and mind are synonymous terms.

There are two senses in which this opinion may be held. It has been maintained by some writers that only what is in the field of consciousness at any present moment is truly mental and that when a presentation passes out of the field of consciousness it passes liter-ally " out of mind." By these writers the problem of mental retention is solved by supposing that the " memory-traces," whose existence we must assume in order to account for conscious recollection, persist in the form of " brain-traces," which have no mental counter-part until they are again roused to functional activity accompanied by consciousness. On the other hand, when consciousness is used to include the whole mass of psychical manifestations, the totality of the mental processes of the individual, it is implied that there is much in the mind that is not in the conscious field of the moment, but nothing which is not now, or has not at some time been, in consciousness in this strict sense of the word. On this view memory-traces exist as mental-traces or dispositions, and in their latent state as well as in their active state form part of the mind.

In these two senses, then, it has been held that con-sciousness and mind are equivalent. The former view is very commonly held by physiologists. The latter is that which has been held by the majority of psychologists up to recent times.

When those who believe that the passing wave of consciousness alone is truly mental speak of an idea becoming unconscious, they mean that it has no longer any existence except in the form of some physical trace left in the *brain*. And the brain, as material substance, is unconscious in the same sense as inanimate objects are said to be unconscious. If, however, we believe that when an idea passes out of the conscious field it leaves behind a trace or disposition in the *mind*, the total sum of such mental dispositions, so long as they are latent, may be said to form an unconscious part of the mind. And this is a use of the word unconscious which is very commonly made.

So long as cerebral-traces or mental dispositions give no evidence of activity it may be convenient to speak of them as unconscious, if we suppose that so soon as they become active they will manifest in consciousness again. But when evidence is found of the occurrence of mental activity which does not appear in consciousness and cannot be discerned on introspection, the inadequacy of this distinction between conscious and unconscious becomes apparent. The static physical view of unconsciousness—the hypothesis of brain-traces, has to be supplemented by the further hypothesis of some sort of " unconscious cerebration " which is capable of doing mental work without any mental accompaniment ; and, in the alternative view the mental dispositions must be accredited with activity and consciousness in some degree, though not in a degree sufficient to attract the attention and be discerned on introspection.   This latter supposition is the hypothesis of *subconsciousness* as this was first formulated by writers on general psychology.

We know that the field of consciousness has always a focus which is the centre of attention, and that outside this focus there is a margin in which discrimination becomes less and less exact as we recede from the focus ; and the principle of continuity compels us to believe that beyond the margin, also, something of the nature of consciousness exists.   This possibility is commonly described in terms of a psycho-physical threshold which can be overstepped only by such feelings or thoughts as attain a certain degree of intensity ; and such feelings or thoughts as do not attain the necessary intensity are said to be subconscious.

The need for postulating any subconsciousness beyond the margin discernible on introspection was not very keenly felt by psychologists so long as they confined themselves to the study of the normal mind ; but when such facts as those revealed in Janet's investigations of hysteria came to light, it became urgently necessary to find some term by which to describe them.   The dissociated sensations and movements of hysteria were called subconscious by Janet, and it was very commonly supposed that the subconsciousness of such hysterical manifestations was the same kind of subconsciousness as that which has been postulated by some psychologists as existing in every normal mind.   Yet Janet himself has clearly shown that the hysteric's failure to perceive sensory impressions applied to an anæsthetic area is not due to lack of intensity of the modification of consciousness so produced, but to a dissociation whereby these modifications fail to be assimilated to the " personal consciousness." For it is obvious, in his experiments, that there was some sort of awareness of the impressions which was not dim or confused, but was clear and discriminative. The most striking feature of this awareness is that it was an awareness concomitant, though not compresent, with the awareness of the impressions received through other sense organs which were not anæsthetic. There was a kind of consciousness which is best described by Dr. Morton Prince's term " co-consciousness."

The implication of diminished intensity contained in the term subconscious makes the use of this word inadvisable when we wish to refer to such mental activities as those revealed in hysteria and multiple personality. Moreover, by using Dr. Prince's term " co-conscious," we emphasize the important fact that in these dissociations we have an actual splitting of *consciousness*, not merely a splitting of the mind. For we may have dissociation of the mind in which the split-off portion shows no evidence of being accompanied by awareness and seems to be truly unconscious.

It would seem useful to have some other term to describe all that exists or takes place below the threshold of consciousness, whether it be subconscious or co-conscious or unconscious. The word " subliminal " was used by Frederic Myers just in this sense, and it would perhaps be convenient if we could still use it in the sense defined by him. He said : " The idea of a *threshold* (*limen*, *Schwelle*) of consciousness—of a level above which sensation or thought must rise before it can enter into our conscious life—is a simple and familiar one. The word *subliminal*—meaning ' beneath that threshold '—has already been used to define those sensations which are too feeble to be individually recognized. I propose to extend the meaning of the term, so as to make it cover *all* that takes place beneath the ordinary threshold, or say, if preferred, outside the ordinary margin of consciousness—not only those faint stimulations whose very faintness keeps them submerged, but much else which psychology as yet scarcely recognizes ; sensations, thoughts, emotions, which may be strong, definite and independent, but which by the original constitution of our being, seldom emerge into that supraliminal current of consciousness which we habitually identify with ourselves." [1]

It may be seen that the ambiguity, already referred to, pertaining to the use of the word consciousness, follows us here if we try to be clear about the *locus* of this threshold. In the first part of the paragraph quoted above Myers is obviously referring to a threshold which lies between what is in consciousness and what is out of consciousness at the moment ; but in the latter part the threshold seems to separate that part of the mind which is capable of becoming conscious from a part which ordinarily has no such power. It is a threshold between the self that each of us knows by introspection and a hidden self of which we have no direct cognizance.

Between what is conscious at the moment and what is unconscious or subliminal at the moment there is a clear distinction, and it would seem to be urgently necessary to distinguish also between that part of the subliminal which is capable of entering consciousness and the part which is not capable of doing so. Such a distinction has been drawn by Freud. That part of the mind which is out of consciousness at the moment, but

[1] *Human Personality*, Vol. I, p. 14.

is capable of entering into it—the memories of every kind which we have at our disposal—he calls the *preconscious*. That part of the mind which is out of consciousness at the moment and is incapable of entering into it under any ordinary circumstances, he calls the *Unconscious* " proper." Preconscious ideas are latent because for the time being their activity is slight; they are too feeble to step over the threshold of consciousness. But, when they become strong, they overstep the threshold and enter the conscious field. Freud maintains, however, that some ideas, namely, those that are repressed, cannot enter into consciousness, no matter how strong and active they may be. Such ideas he calls Unconscious in the technical sense of the word.

It is perhaps unfortunate that Freud uses the word unconscious both in the descriptive sense of being out of consciousness at the moment, thereby making it include the preconscious, and also in the particular technical sense of the Unconscious proper—the unconscious constituted by repression. This double usage tends to set up a confusion similar to that which accrued from the old custom of using the word consciousness so as to include within it what we now call the preconscious as well as what we may call the conscious " proper." Nevertheless Freud's division of mental process and content into conscious, preconscious and unconscious, makes for clearness and precision when we attempt to give a regional or topographical description of the structure of the mind.

It is not, however, in a descriptive sense only that Freud employs these terms. He uses them also in a " systematic " sense, which is even more significant for his psychological theories. He conceives of the mind as a reflex system—a mental reflex arc—sensory or receptive at one end and motor or executive at the other. Any stimulus applied at the receptive end sets up a movement which tends to spread to the motor end. The setting up of this movement, the initiation of any mental process, is accompanied by release of psychical energy, the accumulation of which is experienced as discomfort. This psychical energy, which corresponds to what Freud calls " affect," must find an outlet, and the goal of the activity set up is to effect the discharge of this energy and thereby to bring the system to a condition of rest again. The state of excitation, which is experienced as discomfort, is thus changed to a state of relief, which is experienced as pleasure, and the tendency within the mind to effect this change is what Freud calls a " wish."

A healthy child, before it is born, may be said to have no wishes. All its needs are gratified continuously so that the state of discomfort never arises. And even after it is born the nurse or mother attends to all its wants. But if some need is felt, if some stimulus occurs which is not immediately nullified by the need being satisfied, the mental process characteristic of a wish is set up. The excitation set up has two courses open to it; namely, forwards towards the motor end, where from the nature of the case no adequate paths can be found, or backwards towards the sensory end, thereby reviving the sensations or perceptions which had on former occasions accompanied gratification of the need—for example, in the case of hunger, the sensation of being fed. When this latter path is followed, the perceptions which accompanied former satisfactions are revived with hallucinatory vividness and the child experiences gratification which for the time being stills the excitement in the mental system. When, however, the craving induced by the need is insistent, as in the case of hunger, the hallucinatory perception soon fails to satisfy, and the excitement within the system presses more urgently towards the motor end of the arc and gives rise to inco-ordinate movements and cries which attract the attention of the nurse or mother so that the child's wants are satisfied.

The chief characteristic of such a mental system is the freedom with which it permits the psychical impulse to spread throughout all its parts in search, as it were, for some outlet for the discharge which would bring the whole system to rest again. When this is achieved, pleasure is experienced, so that the purpose of the movement may be said to be the pursuit of pleasure ; the system is actuated by what Freud calls the " pleasure-principle."

The tendency of the movement set up within the system to regress to the sensory end of the mental arc, thereby affording hallucinatory gratification, is very soon found to be unsuitable to the demands of the " real " world into which the child has come. Therefore a secondary mental system arises, or comes into action, which secures the inhibition of the tendency to regression and directs the impulses towards the motor end of the mental arc so as to bring about, by action upon the external world, the changes necessary for the production of a real perception, a real gratification, instead of an imaginary one. The activity of this secondary system is guided by what Freud calls the " reality-principle," in contradistinction to the pleasure-

5

principle underlying the activities of the primary system.

Just as, in the pursuit of pleasure by the primary system, the tendency to regression is inadequate to reality, so also is the method adopted by this system in the avoidance of pain. It retreats before a painful stimulus and ignores it. There is no tendency to revive the painful memory, but rather to get away from it. But adaptation to the " real " world necessitates that a certain amount of pain must be borne, and painful memories formed, if only for the purpose of securing pleasure and avoiding pain in the future. If the " real " world is to be mastered pain has to be faced, for only by accepting pain as a part of reality is it possible to take any steps to avoid it ; and the avoidance of pain becomes as important an objective for the secondary system as the pursuit of pleasure is for the primary. And here, also, the secondary system secures its end by inhibiting the freedom of movement in the primary system. It makes possible the utilization of memories of painful experience by preventing the development of the pain when the experience is remembered.

Although at first the effect of acting according to the reality-principle appears as an abandonment of the hedonic aims of the primary system in favour of a more utilitarian goal, it may be held, and has been held, that the activities guided by the reality-principle are but a longer way round of securing the same end. The crying of the child when it wants to be fed, thereby attracting the attention of the nurse or mother, is but a roundabout way of achieving a greater satisfaction than was possible by the more direct but less effective path of regression.

The secondary system does but control and guide the energies of the primary system so as to secure more adequately the gratification which the primary system strives for, but achieves only imperfectly because of its want of conformity to reality. So long as they are in agreement as to what is pleasant and what is painful they work harmoniously together. But a time comes when disagreement sets in. With the development of the child's personality it comes to pass that what causes pleasure in the primary system causes pain in the secondary system. The task of the secondary system is here no longer to control and guide the tendencies of the primary system towards a real fulfilment of its wishes. The wishes of the two systems are not now the same. The tendencies which give pleasure to the primary system give pain to the secondary system, and the secondary system tries only to avoid these tendencies and to get away from them. Thus arises a divorce between the two systems which results in the establishment of the mechanism of repression and the formation of the two mental systems which we call the Unconscious and the preconscious.

The primary and secondary systems are thus the forerunners of the Unconscious and the preconscious. The Unconscious retains all the characteristics of the primary system : it is guided solely by the pleasure-principle ; it can do nothing but wish, and in the pursuit of the gratification of its wishes the freest possible movement of the psychic impulses is permitted just as in the primary system. Thus it is found that in the Unconscious the associative bonds capable of linking one idea with another are often of the flimsiest description ; the most superficial resemblances are sufficient to bring together ideas which may appear wholly disparate to the conscious mind. The restrictions of logical thought have here no place and direct contradictions are entirely disregarded. In the preconscious, on the contrary, mental process is subservient to the needs of reality, phantasy thinking is subject to control, and present pleasure is foregone for the sake of future good. Yet just as the secondary system does not always succeed in mastering the tendency to regression, so the preconscious is ever at war with the Unconscious and sometimes becomes subject to its domination. It is the conflict between the primary and secondary mental systems, when the pleasure of the one becomes the pain of the other, that gives rise to the mechanism of repression ; and the earliest repressions thus brought about form the core of the Unconscious throughout life.

The whole of the content of the mind would seem to be divided by Freud into that which, in the systematic sense, is preconscious and that which is unconscious. The content of consciousness is really part of the preconscious system. Consciousness itself he compares to a sense organ which perceives certain processes set up in the preconscious. Some of Freud's disciples have supposed that Freud was the first to make this comparison of consciousness to a sense organ, but it is really a very old notion in psychology. A very similar view may be found in the writings of the Scottish school of philosophers and of their French followers at the beginning of the nineteenth century. Royer-Collard, for example, held that " our sensations, acts, thoughts, pass before our consciousness as the waters of a river under the eye of a spectator on its banks." Consciousness has also been compared to a stage on which plays are acted, but this simile would apply better to that part of the preconscious of which consciousness is the spectator.

Whether or no this comparison of consciousness to a sense organ is legitimate, it is useful in that it emphasizes the fact that neither the contents nor the processes of consciousness have any peculiar characteristics other than those that belong to the preconscious. The preconscious contents are just those that are qualified to enter consciousness, and conscious process and preconscious process have been one from the beginning. On the other hand the contents of the Unconscious are just those contents of the mind that are disqualified from entering consciousness in undisguised form, and unconscious process has been different from preconscious process from the beginning.

Freud does not often use the metaphor of a threshold in delimiting the different regions of the mind, but just as we speak of a threshold between the conscious and the preconscious, so we may say there is a threshold between the preconscious and the Unconscious ; but this threshold has a barrier. The doorway here is not freely open to every idea that is strong enough to overstep the threshold. There appears to be a door-keeper—the Freudian " censor "—who discriminates between the applicants and selects those that may be admitted into the preconscious. The censor has behind him all the repressing forces which keep out of the preconscious those ideas that would be unbearable if they became conscious.

The unconscious due to repression is the Unconscious " proper " or true Unconscious of Freudian psychology. It is that part of the mind which retains the characteristics of the primary system, is guided by the pleasure-principle, and is under repression. The preconscious, on the other hand, is that part of the mind which retains the characteristics of the secondary system, is guided by the reality-principle, and is the source of the repressing forces.

This is the " systematic " meaning of the term unconscious, which in its descriptive meaning of being merely " out of consciousness " includes the preconscious. To say that a thought or mental process is unconscious should, in psycho-analytic writings, be understood to imply that it belongs to that mental system whose mode of functioning belongs to what Freud calls the " primary process " ; but it cannot be said that authors have adhered to this usage, or that the context always makes it clear when it is used in the descriptive and when in the systematic sense.

A further source of confusion is found in the fact that certain preconscious contents which form associative connexions with unconscious contents are subject to repressing forces ; their emergence into consciousness is met with resistance, and they are therefore in the " systematic " sense unconscious. Freud provides for them a second censor, which he places between the conscious and the preconscious.

Freud's explanation of the origin of the Unconscious accords well with the nature of its contents and processes which he discovered by the technical methods of psychoanalysis. As we have seen, he met with great resistance in his patients when he tried to bring back to consciousness the pathogenic memories for which he sought, and he concluded that this resistance was due to the same force—the repression—which had originally caused the forgetting. He also found that when he did succeed in restoring the lost memories their recollection was accompanied by the display of much painful emotion, and that their painfulness seemed to depend on their incompatibility with the moral or æsthetic standards of the patient. His further investigations showed that the unconscious determinants of the neurosis could be traced in every instance to those repressed infantile tendencies which he calls sexual. We are thus prepared to find that the Unconscious consists essentially of just those tendencies or wishes whose satisfaction gives pleasure to the child but would be reprehensible or painful to the adult ; for it is the occurrence of a change in the affective tone pertaining to the gratification of these wishes which originally causes them to be repressed.

And this is indeed the teaching of psycho-analysis. The Unconscious is just the infantile mind, persisting throughout life, covered over, as it were, by the adult mind which has developed in response to the claims of reality. Moreover, this infantile part of the mind is not wholly derived from the childhood of the individual ; it is partly derived from the childhood of the race. And some of the tendencies derived from this latter source have never entered consciousness, even for a moment, but have been under repression from the very beginning. When we realize that the Unconscious is not merely a passive receptacle for repressed memories, but the seat of dynamic energies, we may understand how mental processes may remain for ever unconscious although profoundly influencing life and conduct.

The dynamic and striving nature of the Unconscious is one of its most important characteristics. Another is that it has no moral standards whatsoever, and is

entirely lacking in all the qualities which we ascribe
to our conscious logical thought. It is a-moral and
a-logical, and consequently its desires are always in
conflict with those of the conscious personality.

Such is the nature of the contents and processes of
the true Unconscious of Freudian psychology. The
repressing forces to which its existence is due are derived
from the "ego-tendencies" which provide all the
æsthetic, moral, and logical qualities which have
enabled man to adapt himself to the social world in
which he has to live. The actual forces which cause
and maintain the repression would seem to be exercised
by the affective side of his nature, for it is such emotions
as shame, loathing, disgust, which are regularly found
to accompany the return of the repressed material
when the resistance is overcome.

The arousal of such emotions by the primitive tendencies, when the change in the affective values of these
occurs, is no doubt greatly stimulated by training and
education—especially by manifestations of social disapproval ; but it cannot be supposed that the altered
emotional reactions which supervene when this stage
of development is reached are produced by external
influences alone in the course of the individual life.
We must believe that the readiness so to react is an
inherited function of the preconscious and that its
emergence in the child is part of the recapitulation of
racial history and marks the period of man's transition
from the brute to the human.

If all psychologists accepted Freud's conclusions as
to the origin and nature of the Unconscious, there would
be little room for any considerable ambiguity in the
terms used to delimit the different regions of the mind.

Indeed, if all those who more or less consistently use his technical methods and base their conceptions on the results of mental analysis, could have adhered to his nomenclature, so far as it served their purpose, we should have been saved some of the difficulties which beset our path when we try to correlate the findings of the different schools.

The Zürich school of Analytical Psychology, founded by C. G. Jung, is an offshoot from the psycho-analytic school of Freud. For a considerable number of years Jung supported Freud's teaching and practised his methods; but latterly he has diverged in several directions from the psycho-analytic standpoint. One of the most important of these divergencies concerns the nature and origin of the unconscious.

Jung defines the unconscious as " the totality of all psychic phenomena that lack the quality of consciousness." He says that instead of being called unconscious these phenomena may equally well be called subliminal —a term which, in his view, presupposes the hypothesis that each psychic content must possess a certain energic value in order that it may become conscious. Such an admission would seem to imply that in Jung's view every content of the unconscious is unconscious because it has not sufficient energic value or intensity to overstep the threshold. This would exclude the whole of the true Unconscious of Freud, because an essential characteristic of a psychic content that is unconscious in the " proper " Freudian sense, is that it cannot enter consciousness simply in virtue of its strength or activity. Yet Jung also believes that in addition to all lost memories, and the subliminal associations and combinations of these that may occur, an important part of the unconscious results from "intentional repressions" of painful and incompatible thoughts and feelings.

It is doubtful how far the results of "intentional repression" correspond with those due to the repressing forces which come into play without any conscious intention ; and this latter form of repression is of prime importance in the formation of the Unconscious of Freud. However this may be, Jung explicitly states that the "personal" unconscious contains intentional repressions as well as all lost memories and the subliminal combinations they may form.

He calls these contents of the unconscious "personal" because they are all derived from experience in the individual life and are unique in every person. But he postulates another stratum or form of the unconscious which is not the product of acquisitions during the individual life, but is inherited or innate. It contains the psychic potentialities which are common to every individual, such as the instincts and the congenital conditions of intuition—the "archetypes of apprehension," as he calls them. The sum of these inherited psychic potentialities he calls the "Collective Unconscious," because they are common to all men and not unique individual contents like those which form the personal unconscious.

The collective unconscious is the part or form of the unconscious on which Jung now lays most stress. Here are to be found the instincts which we all have in common —the true determinants of our conscious actions. Here also are those primordial forms of thought and feeling which determine the uniformity of our apprehension of the world. These primordial thought-feelings—for they are feeling as much as thought—form the basis of intuition. Just as the instincts enter into or influence our conscious activities which we believe to be rationally motivated, so these primordial thought-feelings, which represent primeval man's way of apprehending the world, enter into or influence our conscious rational thinking. They are the source of all the myths and legends and religions of humanity, whose similarity amongst all peoples and in all ages is accounted for by their common origin in the collective unconscious of the race. In normal life they come to light in more or less disguised form in dreams ; in the neuroses they press obtrusively on the conscious personality, making difficult that adaptation to reality which is man's chief task ; in the insanities they break through the accretions of ages of culture and civilization and manifest in their primordial forms.

In primitive man, according to Jung, when personal differentiation is only beginning, " his mental function is essentially collective. He is more or less identified with the collective psyche, and therefore without any personal responsibility or inner conflict ; his virtues and vices are collective. Conflict only begins when a conscious personal development of the mind has already started. . . . The repression of the collective psyche, in so far as it was conscious, was a necessity for the development of the personality, because collective psychology and personal psychology are in a certain sense irreconcilable . . . a collective point of view, although it may be necessary, is always dangerous for the individual." [1]

It is interesting to compare the factors in this repres-

[1] *Analytical Psychology*, p. 453.

sion of the collective unconscious with those involved in the repression of the primitive impulses as described by Freud. The opposition between society and the individual is present in both ; but the collective is repressed because it is dangerous to the development of the individual ; the primitive impulses are repressed because they are dangerous to the development of society. Repression of the collective is a reaction of the individual against the encroachments of the social consciousness ; repression of the impulses is due to a reaction of the social consciousness against the ego centric tendencies of the individual.

In Freud's psychology the two great subdivisions of the mind are the preconscious and the unconscious. In the psychology of Jung a similar importance is ascribed to what is personal and what is impersonal or collective. The conscious contents as well as the unconscious contents are partly personal and partly impersonal. " The unconscious contents are partly personal, in so far as they concern solely repressed materials of a personal nature, that have once been relatively conscious and whose universal validity is therefore not recognized when they are made conscious ; partly impersonal in so far as the materials concerned are recognized as impersonal and of a purely universal validity, of whose earlier even relative consciousness we have no means of proof." [1]

It is evident that the different bases of classification of the contents of the mind employed by Freud and Jung lead to cross-divisions, so that it is difficult to be sure in what division of the one classification any particular content in the other should be placed. The

[1] *Analytical Psychology*, p. 472.

true Unconscious of Freud would seem to correspond in many respects to the impersonal or collective unconscious of Jung, for the primitive impulses which form the core of the Freudian Unconscious, and the primary process which it retains as its mode of functioning, must be deemed to have universal validity, since they are common to all mankind. In so far, however, as the primitive impulses acquire individual differentiation in infancy, they must be regarded as pertaining to the personal unconscious. But in the true Unconscious of Freud, as in the collective unconscious of Jung, is to be sought the origin of unconscious phantasies, of the language of the dream, and of the myths and legends of humanity.

Although at first sight there may not seem to be any serious incompatibility between the two views, yet we know they form the foundations on which have been built up two systems of psychopathology and psychotherapeutics which, although they had a common origin, have diverged so much that they seem to be pointing in opposite directions. The differences between the two schools cannot be said to be wholly due to differences about the nature of the unconscious ; but some of them are directly dependent upon these, and only in so far as we may find common ground between the two views of the unconscious can we expect to find any common outlook on therapeutic problems and aims.

The Freudian view of the Unconscious is more definite and precise than that of the Swiss school. It is just the infantile mind, still subject to the primary process, and still striving for the gratification of the primitive impulses. Complicating this simplicity, however, is the fact that preconscious contents may fall under the sway of unconscious wishes, and, being thereby charged with the affective tone of the Unconscious, become subject to a censorship which prevents their emergence into consciousness. Notwithstanding this possibility and its far-reaching consequences, we may still feel it hard to believe that everything in the mind that cannot enter consciousness is under direct or indirect repression. This difficulty is especially acute when we consider the creative side of mental activity. We get here the impression—conforming to Jung's view—that some things do not enter into consciousness because they are not yet ready or ripe to do so. Presumably such ideas belong to the preconscious system, and their non-emergence into consciousness is due to a lack of the intensity necessary to enable them to cross the threshold. But when we survey the whole field of man's mental activity, and take cognizance of those of its products which show signs of subliminal incubation, we may sometimes be in doubt concerning the regional localization of processes which, in the descriptive, if not in the systematic sense, are unconscious.

CHAPTER V

PSYCHO-ANALYSIS

(a) PSYCHO-ANALYSIS AS A PSYCHOLOGICAL METHOD

PSYCHO-ANALYSIS is a method of investigating the contents and processes of the human mind. Like all other methods that are of any value it is based ultimately upon introspection. Only by introspection do we have any direct knowledge of mind, even the experimental method having to depend, for the interpretation of its data, upon the experimenter's knowledge of what goes on in his own mind. Apart from introspection and experiment the most important source of knowledge of mind is found in the products of mental activity in others when these are revealed by outward signs such as the expression of the emotions or behaviour as a whole. An extension of this indirect method is its application to the products of man's mind which are embodied in his language, his literature, his art, and in his institutions, laws and religions. This objective method is also necessarily employed in genetic psychology and in comparative psychology—the psychology of animals, of infancy, of peoples and of abnormal individuals. But here, again, it must be emphasized that introspection is the necessary foundation underlying all interpretation of what is observed. We can reconstruct the feelings and thoughts of others only

through the interpretation of the external manifestations of such feelings and thoughts by analogy with
what we discover in our own minds.

This consideration is of peculiar significance for the
estimate we may form of psycho-analysis as a method
of psychology. For psycho-analysis is one of the
indirect methods whose validity depends on the interpretation of our observations in the light of what we
know by introspection ; and the object of psycho-
analytic investigation being the unconscious contents
and processes of the minds of others, our understanding
of what we discover, and, indeed, our ability to discover
anything, will depend on how much we know directly
of similar contents and processes in our own minds.
But these, by definition, are unconscious and are not
normally open to introspection, so that the method of
psycho-analysis is beset by an inherent difficulty which
is not encountered in any other psychological method.
It is true that our ordinary powers of introspection have
to be trained in order that they may be useful in psychological investigation, but they are powers which
every one has in a greater or less degree. Ability to
perceive one's own Unconscious, however, is not an
everyday possession, and very special means are necessary in order to develop it. Thus it has come to be
realized that no one is fully capable of conducting a
psycho-analysis unless he has first of all submitted his
own mind to a similar process. Only by so doing can
he attain the clearness of mental vision which is need-
ful for penetrating the dark regions of the Unconscious.
To some extent this may be achieved by self-analysis :
were it otherwise, the method of psycho-analysis could
never have been discovered ; but for most people the

resistances against such self-knowledge as analysis implies are too great to be overcome unaided.

Psycho-analysis may be said to have originated when Freud discarded hypnotism as a means of broadening the field of consciousness, and decided to seek some other way of recovering the forgotten memories of his patients. As has been briefly indicated in a previous chapter, his first attempts at doing so took the form which he called the "pressure method." He assured the patient that the correct memory would emerge when he pressed his hand on the patient's forehead. Only occasionally, however, could the sought-for memories be evoked directly in this way. Most frequently the ideas which arose seemed to be irrelevant and were rejected by the patients themselves as being incorrect. But Freud was deeply imbued with the belief that in the mental world, as in the physical, nothing can happen without a cause and that every psychical process must be as strictly determined by its antecedents as are the events with which physical science has to deal. He therefore thought that if the patient set out with the intention of recalling some forgotten experience, no idea that came to consciousness during his search could be wholly unconnected with what he was seeking.

But besides the conscious intention of the patient to recall the lost memory, another force had to be reckoned with, namely, that opposing force which was experienced as resistance. And it soon became clear that the greater the resistance the less evident was the connexion between the emergent idea and the sought-for memory. Yet it was found that there was always *some* connexion between the two. If the resistance was slight the lost memory might emerge in undisguised form ; but if resistance was great, the idea which appeared merely pointed the way to the repressed memory by alluding to it in some indirect manner.   When the hints thus afforded were patiently and perseveringly followed up, the pressure method would often succeed in bringing to consciousness the repressed ideas and feelings which had given rise to the symptoms.

At first Freud followed the plan adopted by Breuer and set out to find the lost memories related to some particular symptom ; but when the complex structure of even the simplest neurosis came to be realized, the practice of starting from an individual symptom, with the object of discovering its origin, was abandoned. It was found that nothing less than analysis of the whole mental structure of the neurosis was necessary, and instead of beginning the analysis with the symptom as a starting-point, it became customary to allow the patient to begin wherever he liked, the only injunction being that he should relate whatever came into his mind without exercising any selection or criticism of the incoming thoughts.   The one initial idea from which he set out was his desire to get well, and Freud believed that, with this as a starting-point, if the patient uttered freely everything that occurred to him, nothing that he said could be irrelevant.

In this method all voluntary direction of thought has to be avoided and one idea must be allowed to call up another without question or criticism. Nothing is to be left unsaid because of its unpleasantness or seeming irrelevance, and the mind must be allowed to run as freely as possible—as freely as the resistances permit. This way of conducting analysis is known as the method of " free association," and it remains to the present day the most characteristic and important feature of psycho-analytic technique.

In analysis carried out by the method of free association the direct expenditure of force by the analyst, which led Freud to his conceptions of resistance and repression, is to a great extent avoided. Instead of urging the patient to recall memories related to particular symptoms the psycho-analyst of to-day relies on the free association of the patient ; for these associations, he believes, are not really free, but psychically determined, and lead surely if slowly to the forgotten memories. Resistance is not felt now as a psychic force against which the analyst has to struggle, but is revealed by the devious course which the associations take before the proper memories arise.

(b) PSYCHO-ANALYSIS AS A BODY OF DOCTRINE

When we speak of psycho-analysis we may be referring not merely to a special psychological technique or to a therapeutic method but to a particular body of doctrine, relating to the content and process of the mind, which has grown out of the knowledge obtained by this mode of investigation. And just as the psycho-analytic method is mainly concerned with the exploration of the unconscious, so psycho-analytic doctrine emphasizes and elucidates the part played by the unconscious in normal and abnormal mental life.

The most fundamental conceptions of psycho-analytic theory are those that have already been referred to in tracing the origin of the psycho-analytic method, namely, the existence and nature of the unconscious, and the mechanisms by which it comes into being—the mechanisms of conflict and repression. Certain subsidiary conceptions are also an essential part of the superstructure which has arisen on these foundations. Chief among these is the nature of affective processes implied in the hypotheses of conversion and displacement. Important also is the insistence on the dynamic nature of all mental processes and the tracing the source of their energy to the primitive impulses of the instinctive life.

These energies are derived, not only from those instinctive tendencies which reveal themselves throughout life, such as the primary instincts recognized by sociologists and psychologists as underlying and determining most of our conduct ; but also from those tendencies which, owing to their incompatibility with civilized human standards, become repressed and give no direct evidence of their continued existence. This is an essential and characteristic part of psycho-analytic doctrine. The repressed tendencies, although they disappear from conscious life and no longer manifest directly in conduct, are not abolished. They persist in the unconscious, with all their energies unspent, and for these energies some outlet must be obtained.

As we have seen, the primary impulses which are subject to repression belong mainly to that division of infantile activities to which Freud has applied the term sexual. These pleasure-giving activities of childhood are called sexual because analysis of neurotic symptoms leads back to them by way of material which is undoubtedly sexual, and because when they persist into adult life as perversions their sexual character is unhesitatingly recognized by every one.

The motive power behind these infantile activities is ascribed to a striving after pleasure, for at this time they serve no other purpose. They are devoid of any real benefit to the individual, that is, they do not in any way conduce to self-preservation ; and no connexion is as yet established between them and the function of reproduction, although in the course of time those that escape repression become organized under the dominance of the organs of generation and form part of the sexual instinct, in the ordinary acceptance of the term.

The craving for organic satisfaction in the sexual life has long been referred to as *libido*, and in view of the identity of the cravings and the analogy of the satisfactions in childhood and in adult life, Freud has used this term to denote the conative force behind all forms of sexual desire, whether infantile or adult. The main work of psycho-analysis has been the tracing of the life-history of the *libido* through all its ramifications and vicissitudes, as these are presented in neurotic individuals who have submitted themselves to this method of treatment.

The dependence of neurosis upon aberrations in development of the *libido*, and the consequent preoccupation of the psycho-analysts with this topic, have necessarily made it appear as if they had over-emphasized the part played by the sexual instinct in the growth and workings of the mind. They have been accused of denying the importance and extent of other instincts and mental tendencies and of taking a very one-sided view of human nature. In truth, however, they have never denied or forgotten the extent and importance of the *ego-instincts*—as they call those impulses which are opposed to the *libido* and its satisfactions and range themselves on the side of the self which is striving for adaptation to the realities of life. The part played in their doctrines by the conceptions of conflict and repression should alone have prevented misunderstanding on this matter. For if the self possessed no forces stronger than the *libido*-strivings, repression would be impossible. Yet, it is true, the analysts have given us less information about the ego-instincts than about the *libido*, and they confess that they know less about them. Good reason for this is to be found in the nature of the material with which psycho-analysis in the beginning had to deal; but the extension of its application to other conditions besides the psychoneuroses gives promise of enlargement of our knowledge of the ego-impulses and of the relation between the development of personality and the fates of the *libido*-strivings.

From the beginning of the growth of the individual mind, and of the development of the preconscious system, the satisfactions of the *libido* are frustrated by the claims of " reality." The interdictions and training of childhood, the education of later years, intellectual development and the ethical or religious ideals which may be formed, are throughout in conflict with the claims of sexuality whether in infantile or adult forms. The ego-impulses comprise all those forces which are opposed to the *libido*-strivings—all the non-sexual impulses of the personality. But although there are ego-impulses which are distinct from, and opposed to, *libido*-strivings from the beginning—impulses arising mainly in the service of self-preservation—there is also much in the structure of personality, which, though revealing nothing of its sexual origin, can be shown to have arisen from those primary impulses which are repressed in early childhood.

The body of doctrine which has arisen out of psycho-analytic investigation may be said to have been built up from the knowledge, thus obtained, of the fates of these repressed tendencies. Application of psycho-analytic method to the most diverse products and activities of the human mind such as dreams, wit, blunders, neurotic symptoms, traits of character, artistic creations, myths, legends and folk-lore, invariably leads back to unconscious " wishes " and discloses here their source and, in part at least, their explanation.

The normal fate of repressed infantile tendencies— the fate called *sublimation*—is that which is by far the most important ; for on it human progress has depended. Sublimation consists in a displacement of the energies attached to the primitive impulses into channels of activities which are socially acceptable and valuable. We may take as an illustration of the sublimating process the fate of the common childish tendency proudly to display the naked body. In almost all civilized communities gratification of this tendency is regarded as subversive of adult morality and is subject to the repressive forces which are directed against sexuality. Where puritanical standards prevail the tendency of the child may be harshly interdicted, and the shame so aroused may lead to intense repression. But the repressed impulse must find some outlet in adult life ; and this it may do in the self-display that can be effected by means of dress or in other forms of attracting attention. It may be an important factor in the success of the actor, the orator, or the preacher.

The capacity for sublimation seems to have definite limits in each individual. If the repression is too great, or if too much is repressed, sublimation may fail to keep

pace with it ;   and when this is the case, the unsublim-
ated portion of the *libido* will seek out some other mode
of manifestation.   Not much can be done directly to
assist sublimation.   It is essentially an unconscious
process and takes place automatically when suitable
opportunity presents itself.   All we can do is to provide
as many favourable circumstances as possible ; but the
particular form that sublimation may take must be
chosen by the child himself—it cannot be forced upon
him from without.   Particular tendencies can be sublimated only in ways which resemble, or have analogies
with, the ways in which the primitive tendencies manifest themselves.   But the analogy must be one which
appeals to the child's own mind, and cannot be chosen
for him by anyone else.   To the child the new activity
must in some way symbolize or stand for the old activity,
so that the energy belonging to the latter may be transferred to the former : unless it does so the energy will
not flow into the new channels.   Thus, for example, the
educator of the child with exhibitionist tendencies will
fail to assist their sublimation by setting him to play
with bricks or to make mud-pies ; while if he allows
and encourages the instinct of self-display in ways that
are permissible, he may help towards the development
of a great actor or preacher.   Playing with bricks and
making mud-pies are substitute activities for primitive
tendencies of another kind and may lead to greatness
in other paths of life.

Such is the normal fate of a repressed infantile tendency when suitable opportunities for sublimation have
been available.   But in many cases, sublimation is
inadequate, or faulty, and, for one reason or another,
it may sometimes fail completely.   The fate of a repressed

tendency and the issue of the conflict between it and the repressing forces depend upon various circumstances. Satisfactory sublimation is most likely when the strength of the infantile tendency is not too great, when the repressing forces are not too severe, and when suitable opportunities for sublimation are afforded.

Although sublimation, more or less complete, is the normal or usual fate of the primitive tendencies which are subjected to repression, there are other possible fates which are often observed. Sometimes the primitive tendency is so strong from the beginning, or has been allowed or encouraged to become so strong, that the repressing forces may fail. Instead of being repressed the tendency persists, or reappears later in life, as a *perversion*. A sexual perversion is just the persistence into adult life of such infantile tendencies : the child who loves to display the body becomes an exhibitionist.

When the repressing forces are too great a totally different result may ensue. Instead of the persistence of the tendency, a strong *reaction* against it may take place ; and the adult character may then show traits which are the extreme opposite of the unconscious tendency. In this case the child who loves self-display may develop a bashfulness and shrinking self-consciousness which makes life a burden, or may grow into a prude who deprecates the nude in art and sees indecency in every evening frock.

A third possibility, when sublimation fails, is the development of a *nervous illness*. Here the strength of the repressed tendency and the strength of the repression are so great, and so evenly balanced, that the outcome of the conflict is a compromise in which each of the opposing forces obtains some satisfaction. The neurotic symptom affords a surrogate satisfaction to the unconscious wish, while the repression is gratified by having so distorted the wish that its fulfilment in the symptom is not recognized, and by turning its fulfilment into a punishment.

The life-history of the *libido* reveals two aspects of sexuality which are of equal importance. On the one hand it shows the process of development of the sexual organization from the infantile phase in which the primitive tendencies seek gratification independently of one another, to the adult form in which these tendencies are organized under the dominance of the organs of generation and are subordinated to the function of reproduction. On the other hand it recounts the changes which occur in the selection of the objects towards which the *libido* is successively directed, and the consequences of the attachments which may thereby be formed.

The sexual organization of the child and its relation to the sexual perversions have already been briefly indicated in so far as perversion is an aberration in the development of the sexual aim. The sexual aims of childhood are the gratifications of the individual tendencies, any one of which may be as powerful as another. In the perversions one of these primitive tendencies persists as the chief bearer of the *libido*, and the others are subjected to its dominance and utilized in its service. But its aim is an infantile one, and since it is dissociated from the function of reproduction and is pursued only for the sake of pleasure, it is rightly regarded as perverse. There are, however, other aberrations in the development of the sexual life, in which the abnormality consists in the nature of the object towards which the *libido* is directed rather than in the kind of action to which it impels.

The *libido* may be described as attaching itself to, or " investing " or being " occupied with," the objects from which it obtains gratification. In infancy the child gets auto-erotic satisfaction in various ways from the erotogenic zones of its own body, and this leads to the self or ego becoming the object of the *libido*. To this phase of *libido*-development the term *narcissism* is applied, for it corresponds to a perversion of the same name in which all the affection ordinarily given to another is directed towards a person's own body. Like Narcissus he falls in love with himself.

The narcissistic phase in the life of the *libido* normally gives place very soon to object-love, properly so called, in which the *libido* flows out towards the external world and becomes attached to those persons or things from which the desired satisfactions can be obtained. But not all of the narcissistic *libido* is thus transformed. A certain residue is always left behind so that a certain amount of self-love is common to every one. And when any object becomes invested with *libido* such object tends to be overestimated, so that when the imperfections of the self revealed by dawning self-knowledge come to be realized, the narcissistic *libido* may become displaced on to the ideal of the self which is formed in the course of social and ethical education and culture. The construction of an ideal self towards which the *libido* can be directed re-establishes the satisfaction derived from the infantile narcissism and forms some compensation for the disillusionment which life so easily brings regarding the true value and importance of one's own personality. Idealization is thus seen to be a deflection of narcissistic *libido* which has something in common with the deflection of object-libido in sublimation. But the two processes are not entirely analogous. For in sublimation there is a deflection of the *libido* towards a goal which is no longer sexual : in idealization there is merely a different way of looking at an object which still retains its sexual character.

At the beginning of the phase of true object-love, when auto-erotism is given up, the *libido* is turned towards the mother. The mother is the first real love-object. Towards her the tender emotion which forms the psychical side of the sexual life is first emphasized. And when this takes place repression of the physical side of love—the merely sensual gratification of the impulses—has already begun, so that the way is paved for that " incestuous " fixation of the *libido* on the parents which gives rise to what is known as the " Œdipus Complex." The affection of the small boy for the mother and of the girl for the father, the preferences and the jealousies which they show, are not solely due to the egoistic satisfactions afforded by the care and attention bestowed by the parents. They also contain an erotic or sensual element, as indeed do also the preferences of each parent for the children of the opposite sex. The evidence in support of this view cannot be entered upon here, but it must be understood that the part played by the family attachments in the growth and structure of personality is the very core of the body of doctrine which has grown out of psychoanalytic investigation.

The first love-object of humanity is thus always an incestuous one. The *libido*, at first directed towards the parents, may later be displaced on to brothers or sisters, and since the sexual implications of love tend to be more and more realized as the child grows older, so repression of the incestuous *libido* becomes more and more intense. But the fixation of the *libido* on incestuous objects in the unconscious is incompatible with a normal life in later years, and one of the great tasks of every human being is to free the *libido* from its unconscious attachments to the family and to direct it towards some suitable object in the outer world.

Fixation is the technical term applied to arrest in development of any of the components of the sexual instinct in its progress from the infantile to the adult form ; or to an undue adhesiveness of the *libido* to the incestuous objects of childhood. If excitement of an infantile sexual tendency takes place too early, or if indulgence in the means of securing its gratification is excessive or carried on too long, the *libido* pertaining to these tendencies becomes reluctant to give up this mode of obtaining satisfaction and is arrested or falls behind in the onward progress towards the normal adult sexual organization. And just so far as the total amount of *libido* available is depleted by such early fixation, so, the *libido* which follows the normal development and attains to adult organization is, to the same degree, weakened and thus made less able to overcome the obstructions to its satisfactions which life may present. We know that throughout the whole animal kingdom the sexual goal is not attained without struggle and danger, and in human communities the natural difficulties are reinforced by those imposed by law and custom, morality and religion.

When the *libido*, striving towards satisfaction, meets with opposition which seems too great to be overcome, it tends to turn backwards towards those earlier satisfactions which childhood had afforded. This turning back of the *libido* in the face of external or internal difficulties is known as *regression*. It may be of two kinds : there may be a regression of the *libido* to an earlier phase of sexual organization, such as the infantile phase, before the primacy of the genitals was established, in which the components of the instinct each sought satisfaction in its own way ; or there may be a regression in respect of the objects towards which the *libido* is directed, for example, a return to the incestuous objects of childhood. The reanimation of these primitive tendencies by the regressive *libido* and the increased intensity which the unconscious wishes thereby acquire, are the immediate cause of that partial failure of repression which leads to neurosis.

The fates of the *libido* in the course of its history, both in respect of its organization and of its objects, form the main topics of psycho-analytic investigation and provide the basis for the main tenets of psycho-analytic doctrine. These fates are so various, the possibilities of successful sublimation and the consequences of aberrant development are so momentous, that even the imperfect knowledge of them already attained throws light on more than half of human life.

(c) Psycho-analysis as a Therapeutic Instrument

The technique of psycho-analysis was devised, and the most far-reaching of the theories based upon its employment were formulated, under the pressure of the practical motive of relieving the disabilities of neurotic patients ; and although its principles and methods have been applied with very fruitful results to other products of mental activity and in other spheres of interest, psychopathology and psychotherapeutics are still the most important sources of our advancing knowledge.

The success of psycho-analysis as a method of treatment is not, however, the chief ground for its claims on our attention as a topic of importance in the Psychology of Medicine. Of more scientific interest, though of less immediate utility, is the flood of light which it has shed on the mechanism of nervous and mental disorders. Many of these are uninfluenced by psycho-analytic treatment carried out with our present technique ; but it is permissible to hope that the fuller knowledge we now have and are still acquiring of the psychological mechanism of these conditions and of the reasons why they remain uncured by analysis, may enable us to devise new methods or refinements of technique which may some day prove effective.

The immediate object of therapeutic analysis is to bring into consciousness the unconscious wishes which through conflict and displacement or conversion have given rise to neurotic symptoms. The main difficulty in accomplishing this is caused by the resistances due to the repressing forces, and the chief task of the analyst is to discover these resistances and to overcome them. When this is done the unconscious thoughts emerge into consciousness and, their accompanying affects being allowed full play, become assimilated by, and subjected to the control of the whole personality.

Although the method of free association persistently applied, combined with the motive provided by the patient's desire to get well, is by itself theoretically adequate to bring to light the unconscious complexes which underlie the neurosis, it is desirable to lay hold of any means that will aid in the analysis and shorten the treatment. And since it is found that some products of mental functioning emerge more directly from the unconscious than do others, it may be readily understood that analysis of such material proves the shortest route into the hidden depths of the mind. Slips of the tongue or pen, mistakes and blunders in everyday life, momentary forgetfulness of things, mannerisms and tricks of speech or movement, actions performed " automatically " when we are said to be preoccupied, errors of omission and commission, and other occurrences of a similar kind—all may be made use of in analysis to disclose unconscious wishes or tendencies which the patient is unwilling to recognize. But the most important of the mental products which come more or less directly from the unconscious is the dream ; and so it happens that much of the work in therapeutic analysis is concerned with the analysis of the patient's dreams. To this topic the following chapter will be devoted

CHAPTER VI

DREAMS

THE importance ascribed to the study of dreams is one of the most striking features of psychopathological research in recent years. Formerly regarded as a fortuitous product of uncontrolled cerebral activity, having no meaning or significance, the dream is now known to be a complex mental structure, fashioned by determinate forces, which half conceals and half reveals the most intimate secrets of the dreamer's personality. These intimate secrets are not merely things that we have hidden from our fellows, but significant tendencies or desires which we have somehow succeeded in keeping hidden from ourselves. The dream is now held, by almost every school of psychopathology, to be a disguised or distorted revelation of what is taking place in the unconscious. By certain technical methods the disguise may be penetrated and the unconscious thoughts from which the dream has arisen may be unmasked. As we have seen, there is considerable difference of opinion concerning what goes on in the unconscious, and this difference has, in great part, arisen from differences in the ways in which dreams have been interpreted.

That dreams have some meaning is a notion which has always appealed to one side of man's nature, and the practice of dream-interpretation has existed in all ages ; but even before the rise of the scientific era it had fallen into disrepute, and, in the end, it was relegated to the domain of occultism and superstition, from which it was rescued by Freud's epoch-making researches. Whatever our ultimate view of the meaning and significance of dreams may be, the foundations of our knowledge must always rest on Freud's pioneer work, and no study of dream life can be usefully undertaken without familiarity with the methods and conclusions of Psychoanalysis.

In trying to understand Freud's views it is important to keep clearly in mind his distinction between the manifest content of the dream and the latent dream thoughts. The manifest content is the dream as it is remembered by the dreamer on awaking ; the latent dream thoughts are the unconscious thoughts revealed by analysis. The manifest content of the dream is often so bizarre and so devoid of any intelligible meaning that there have always been writers who maintain that it is a product of the uncontrolled association of ideas roused by sensory stimuli affecting the body during sleep ; and since all the main incidents of a dream may often be traced to occurrences in the recent life of the dreamer, the establishment of such a connexion is thought to afford all the explanation that is possible or necessary. The views of those writers who make use of analytical methods are quite different from this. While admitting the part played by sensory stimuli, recent perceptions and forgotten memories, they believe that these are brought into the service of unconscious tendencies or desires, and that the dream, as a whole, is a mental structure which, if rightly understood, may be seen to be of profound significance. According to Freud it reveals the presence of unconscious tendencies which have been repressed because they are unacceptable to consciousness ; according to Jung and others of the post-Freudian school, it points the way to lines of conduct that are desirable if the full development of the personality is to be attained and its potential aspirations made manifest.

The Freudian view of the nature of dream and the part it plays in life is most readily understood by examining the dreams of children under five years of age ; for in these there is no disguise, and the latent thought and the manifest content are one. The only difference is that the latent content is a thought, while the manifest content is that thought translated into hallucinatory experience. Some happening of the previous day has left a longing or unfulfilled desire. A small boy is told that he cannot go to the circus to-day, but that he will be taken to-morrow. When he goes to sleep at night the frustrated desire and his interest in the world tend to return and to disturb his slumber. But the child is tired and wants also to continue sleeping. A compromise between the two wishes is effected ; he dreams he is at the circus, and he remains asleep.

It is plain that such a dream is not a meaningless product of haphazard working of the mind. There is no distortion or disguise about it. It is the fulfilment of a wish—a fulfilment in hallucinatory form which, by stilling the psychic stimulus which threatens to disturb sleep, obviates the need for awakening. The dream is thus the guardian of sleep. It arises from a wish which threatens to disturb sleep, and its content being the fulfilment of this wish, sleep is maintained unbroken.

Most of the features of the dreams of children, which anyone can discover without any analysis and without the use of any technical methods, are believed by Freud to pertain to almost all the dreams of adults ; the one noticeable difference being that the true dream thoughts of the adult are always more or less distorted and disguised in the manifest content known to the dreamer. But the adult dream, like the dream of the child, is a meaningful mental product ; it has its origin in some experience of the previous day from which interest has not been wholly withdrawn ; it is a compromise between the desire to sleep and the fulfilment of a wish ; it is a hallucinatory fulfilment of the wish ; it is the guardian of sleep.

The absence of disguise, so characteristic of the dreams of children, is met with in adult dreams when the sleep-disturbing stimulus comes from organic needs, such as hunger or thirst. The hungry man may dream of eating ; the thirsty man may, in his sleep, succeed for a time in allaying his cravings by drinking hallucinatory draughts of water. So, also, the infantile type of dream may occur in adults when impatience to attain some end is strong, or when comfort or assurance is sought. But, apart from these dreams of infantile type, the dreams of adults show such distortion of the latent dream thoughts that their meaning cannot be found without some process of interpretation. The chief method made use of in the interpretation of dreams is the method of free association—the method *par excellence* of psycho-analysis. Another method, necessary when associations are not forthcoming, or when they are forced and irrelevant, is the symbolic interpretation of certain elements in the dream. Only by a combination of these two methods can the full interpretation of any dream be achieved.

The need for these two methods of dream interpretation is due to the fact that there are two separate sources of the distortion which the true dream thoughts undergo in their translation from the latent into the manifest content. Emanating as they do from the unconscious, the dream thoughts contain something which is unacceptable to the conscious personality. Their emergence into consciousness in waking life is prevented by the repressing forces ; but in sleep these forces are somewhat weakened, so that an opportunity to enter consciousness is afforded to the unconscious wishes. But if these objectionable wishes do enter consciousness the sleeper awakes, and it is only because the repressing forces are still sufficiently active to enforce distortion on the incoming thoughts, though not sufficiently strong entirely to exclude them, that the continuation of sleep becomes possible. The forces of repression, active in the production of dream distortion, have been given a special name. They are called the " dream censorship " because they perform a censor's function in that they allow to pass into consciousness only that of which the personality does not too strongly disapprove ; and this they do by means of various mechanisms which lead to distortion of the elements out of which the dream is composed. The process by which the latent thoughts are translated into the manifest content is called *dream-making* or *dream-construction*, the process by which the manifest content is translated back into the latent thoughts is *dream-interpretation*.

In analysing a dream by the method of free association the different parts of the manifest content are taken one by one as starting points for the dreamer's associations. A single element in the manifest content may lead to a wealth of associations, and when these are examined it will be found that in the dream content remembered by the dreamer a *condensation* of the latent thoughts which they represent has been effected. Sometimes certain parts of the latent content are entirely omitted, or only fragments of it are represented in the manifest content ; but the most common form of condensation is that which is effected by fusing together latent elements having something in common, after the fashion of a "composite photograph." Thus many elements in the latent content may be represented by a single element in the manifest content ; and so it comes about that the true dream thoughts are usually much more extensive than the dream as remembered would indicate. This process of condensation is one of the ways by which disguise of the true dream thoughts is effected.

Another mechanism at work in the dream-making is known as *displacement*. This shows itself in two forms. A latent element may be represented by some indirect allusion, such as would not occur to the waking consciousness of the dreamer as a suitable substitute for the thought to which it refers. Displacement may likewise take the form of a change of emphasis, so that the most important element in the latent content may occupy a quite subsidiary position in the manifest content ; or the chief affect in the dream may be attached to elements in the manifest content which represent latent elements to which this affect does not rightly belong.

One of the most constant sources of dream disguise

is the translation of the dream thoughts into *visual images*. The use of words in thinking was a late development in the evolution of mind, and must have been preceded by a thinking in images—the memory images of sensory impressions. The dream-making brings about a regression of the latent thoughts to the crude sensory material out of which they have grown, and it is mainly a regression to visual images. The dramatic character of dreams is due to this, as is also much of the distortion or disguise which the dream presents. But not all thoughts are or can be represented in visual imagery. Abstract thoughts and the thought relationships denoted by such parts of speech as particles and conjunctions are difficult or impossible to depict in sensory imagery, so we are not surprised to find that the relationships denoted by such words as because, therefore, but, etc., are not represented in the manifest dream content, and in dream interpretation have to be supplied according to the nature of the context.

Another peculiarity of primitive thought is the close association which became established in the mind between "opposites." So pronounced was this that in the beginnings of speech the same word was often used to represent two opposed ideas. Evidence of this is to be found on examining the root-words of languages, both ancient and modern. This peculiarity of primitive thought is reverted to in the dream-making, so that a given thought in the latent content may be represented by its opposite in the manifest content. A similar form of the dream-making mechanism is shown in the inversion of the actual content of the dream, so that, as Freud says, in a dream it is often the hare that shoots the sportsman.

All these distorting expedients are due to the activities of the " dream censor," and these activities do not cease with the actual dreaming of the dream. In our efforts to remember a dream the censorship is still at work, and often succeeds in making us believe the dream to have been more unified and coherent than it really was. To this process is given the name of *secondary elaboration*. It is the last of the four great distorting mechanisms employed by the dream censorship—condensation, displacement, dramatization (visual imagery), and secondary elaboration.

But, as has been said, not all the disguise of the true dream thoughts is due to the direct action of the censor. Some of it is due to a peculiarity of unconscious thinking which provides that the thoughts of the Unconscious are already sufficiently distorted to evade the censor, or to be permitted to pass into the consciousness of the dreamer without any further disguise. This second source of distortion or disguise in the manifest content is the " thinking in symbols " which is a permanent attribute of the Unconscious. Certain thought relationships, identification of unlike objects because of some perceived similarity, and the knowledge implicit in symbol formation seem to be common to every human mind ; and when the thoughts of the *Unconscious* enter consciousness during sleep, they do so in that symbolic guise which is the every-day language of the Unconscious. They are admitted without further distortion, in the form of symbols whose significance is not appreciated by the consciousness of the dreamer. *Preconscious* thoughts which have fallen under the sway of unconscious wishes, and so entered into the structure of the dream, are afforded no such facilitation, and it is these thoughts that, in the course of the dream-making, have to be subjected to the distorting mechanisms of condensation, displacement and dramatization.

In the occurrence of dream symbolism, as in regression to visual imagery and to the use of " opposites " and " inversions " in the making of the dream, we have an indication of the archaic character of much of the dream material which needs interpretation. And the interpretation of dream symbols is not possible by the method of free association. The associations which would lead to the discovery of their meaning have not been formed in the life of the individual ; they were formed in some far back period of the history of the race. Therefore the analyst cannot come to their meaning through the associations of the dreamer ; he must supply it from his own knowledge of symbolism derived from other sources. Here again the origins of language, the structure of folk-lore, myth and fairy tales, and the customs and beliefs of primitive peoples give us the key to much in the dream that would otherwise be unintelligible.

Symbolism is thus the second great source of the disguise met with in the manifest content of the dream. It is a form of disguise, not due to the activity of the censor—the work of the repressing forces in the present —but belonging already to the unconscious thoughts. The censor's work is lightened by its presence, and the symbol is freely admitted into the dream because its meaning is unknown to the consciousness of the dreamer.

The wish-fulfilment observed in the dreams of children is the undisguised hallucinatory gratification of wishes which have been in consciousness. But when the distorted dreams of adults represent the fulfilment of wishes they are wishes which are unacceptable to consciousness and must therefore be disguised before they are admitted thereto. The adult dream is, as a rule, the disguised fulfilment of a repressed wish. The objections commonly made to the wish-fulfilment theory of dreams generally show misunderstanding or forgetfulness of what the theory really is. " How can that be the fulfilment of a wish ? " the sceptic asks, when he has related a dream in which there is either no appearance of any wish being fulfilled, or there is some happening which he says is " the last thing I should wish." One has to keep reminding the critic of dream-interpretation, that it is not the dream as remembered by the dreamer which shows wish-fulfilment, but the dream when interpreted. It is especially difficult to convince him that a dream which is accompanied by painful emotion, or by fear, can in any sense be a fulfilment of a wish. And sometimes the objection has some grounds ; for the dream-making may be unsuccessful in effecting a wish fulfilment out of the painful material with which it has to work, and the painful emotions pass over into the manifest content. These cases apart, however, it may naturally be thought that if a wish is gratified it should be accompanied by pleasure, not by pain ; so that the experience of fear or other painful emotion would seem to preclude the possibility of wish-fulfilment. The answer to this difficulty may be found in calling to mind the relation of the dreamer to his unconscious wishes. These wishes are unconscious just because their appearance in consciousness would cause him pain. This is the principle at work in the mechanism of repression, as described in Chapter III. We should suppose therefore that when painful emotions or fear are prominent in a dream it may be that unconscious wishes are being gratified without being sufficiently disguised. And this is what very commonly occurs in those dreams which are known as "anxiety dreams." In anxiety dreams the repressed wish has come too plainly into the dream consciousness, or is about to do so, and the failure of the censor is signalized by the appearance of anxiety and the awaking of the sleeper.

Another type of dream in which it is not at first sight easy to see wish-fulfilment is that which is known as punishment dreams. A dream of this kind is recorded by Freud from his own experience. After he had become famous as a psycho-analyst he sometimes dreamt that he was back in the chemical laboratory where, in his youth, he had wasted much time in unsuccessful chemical analysis. He was rather ashamed of this part of his life, and disliked thinking about it. When he tended to get too proud or boastful of his success in psycho-analysis, this dream would hold up to him, by way of punishment, those other unsuccessful analyses of which he had no reason to be proud. Freud says that here the wish fulfilled belongs to the repressing forces.[1]

There is, however, one class of dream, in which no wish seems to be operative ; there is rather a tendency of the mind to revert in sleep to some significant past experience, generally of a painful character. The battle-dreams so common among soldiers during the war are good examples of this kind of dream. Here the dream

[1] This would seem to be a departure from the original wish fulfilment theory in which *repressed* desire was held to be the driving force behind all dream manifestations. Punishment dreams would seem to conform, rather, to Jung's view of the compensatory or corrective function of the unconscious (see p. 110).

seems merely to repeat some terrible experience, and it is doubtful if there is any hidden wish behind it. Freud has come to believe that this tendency to revert to significant experience is inherent in the mind and is perhaps deeper and more primordial than the pleasure-principle.

The wish fulfilled in most adult dreams is a wish belonging to the true Unconscious and possesses the attributes which belong to this region of the mind ; that is to say, it is instinctive, infantile, sexual, and repressed. This is the unconscious element which is added to the latent dream thoughts derived from the preconscious, and it provides the dynamic force against which the censor has to struggle. Out of the conflict the dream arises. It is because an unconscious wish has become associated with certain thoughts of the day, from which interest has not been wholly withdrawn on going to sleep, that the dream-making is possible ; and the unconscious wish utilizes this material from the preconscious for the purpose of securing its own gratification. The latent thoughts revealed in dream interpretation are therefore often far removed from infantile tendencies. They are of the same nature as those presented by the conscious thinking of the dreamer. They may be reflexions or forebodings, hopes or aspirations ; for preconscious thoughts are concerned with the same problems as present themselves in conscious thinking.

Because these preconscious elements of the latent content come to light in the process of interpretation, it is sometimes maintained that the dream has other purposes besides the fulfilment of unconscious wishes, and other functions besides the preservation of sleep. Maeder, of Zürich, was the first to insist that the dream is occupied with the dreamer's current problems and must be interpreted as an unconscious effort at adjustment of the difficulties of his life. The dream, according to Maeder, is not primarily concerned with reminiscences or with the gratification of repressed wishes, but has a prospective tendency and points towards the future. Silberer believes every dream can be interpreted in at least two different ways—one the psycho-analytic way of Freud, the other the anagogic way in which the infantile wish tendencies are ignored and higher psychic functions of mystical import are brought to light. Both of these points of view are embodied in the method of dream interpretation adopted by Jung, who in his prospective interpretation lays great stress on the myth themes to be found in dreams, and on their importance as guides for the future development of the dreamer's personality.

Maeder, Silberer and Jung are leaders of the post-Freudian school of analysis which has grown up in ways that, as time goes on, diverge further and further from the psycho-analytic standpoint. The lines of thought peculiar to this school have been developed by Jung in particular in their bearings on psychotherapeutics and the psychology of medicine ; and an examination of his treatment of the dream, its functions and its mechanism, reveals the nature of the assumptions on which the analytical psychology of post-Freudians is based.

The dream, in Jung's view, is a revival during sleep of a form of psychical activity which was at one time the only form of thinking of which man was capable. But only in its form—in its language—is the dream archaic ; its content is not concerned with primitive or infantile impulses, but with the dreamer's problems in the present.   In his attempt to adapt himself to life there are points of view, feelings and tendencies potential in his nature which, owing to neglect, or because of repression, have not received due consideration in his conscious life.   Besides his conscious attitude towards his problems he has also an unconscious one, and this is given expression to in the dream.   Herein, according to Jung, lies the significance of the dream and its value in psychotherapeutics.

But although the dreamer's unconscious attitude towards his problems comes to the surface in the dream it is not presented in a form that is immediately understood.   The dream has to be interpreted—not because it contains unacceptable wishes which have been distorted by a " censor," but because it is couched in a language which is not familiar to the dreamer's conscious personality.   This language is the language of symbolism and phantasy, characteristic of primitive thought, but foreign to our conscious thinking now.   It has, however, remained the language of the unconscious and forms the vehicle for all its more direct expressions—in dreams, in poetry, in the plastic arts, in myth and fairy tales.

Jung thus sees in the dream a manifestation of what he calls the " compensatory function " of the unconscious.   The thoughts and feelings and tendencies which in conscious life are too seldom recognized, come to the surface during sleep, when the conscious thought processes are dissociated or in abeyance.   Such thoughts and feelings and tendencies are unconscious because they have been neglected, and their absence from consciousness entails a one-sided reaction which falls short of the fullest adaptation to life of which the individual is capable.   What is missing from consciousness will be found in the unconscious, and the recovery of the missing portions by the interpretations of dreams should ensure a more adequate adjustment to life and a corresponding freedom from neurotic disabilities. Conscious preoccupation with the problems of life necessitates an outlook on the future, a recognition of the ends to be pursued and a choosing of the means by which they may be attained ; and this prospective tendency of conscious thought is assumed by Jung to pertain also to the unconscious. He is no more satisfied by a purely causal explanation of unconscious thought, such as Freudian psychology demands, than he is willing to accept a deterministic view of man's life and behaviour as a whole. He therefore attributes to the dream the same prospective tendency as that which common sense sees in every conscious thought directed towards some end. The dream portrays the subliminal aspect of the total psychological attitude towards the problem which at the moment confronts the dreamer, and if adaptation is to be satisfactory and free from conflict, this aspect must receive due consideration.

Jung explicitly states that in so regarding the dream he does not deny the validity of Freudian interpretation, but he thinks the associative material brought to light in analysis may be regarded from another point of view and may be measured by a standard different from that which Freud employs. In a general way the method adopted by Jung in the interpretation of dreams is the same as that laid down by Freud ; that is to say, the free associations of the dreamer are made use of, and the information so gained is supplemented by that derived from the symbolism of the dream. In detail, however, there is a wide divergence between the two methods. By Jung the free associations of the dreamer as well as the interpretation of the symbolism of the dream are dealt with from two points of view. In so far as the associations consist of actual reminiscences from the past life, and in so far as the symbols are representatives of real objects, interpretation is said to be on the objective plane ; it is analytical or reductive. When the associations refer to the feelings of the dreamer, when every fragment of the dream is considered as a representative of something in the dreamer himself, and when the symbol is regarded as showing, by means of analogy, the forward strivings of the unconscious towards something higher than the conscious personality has yet attained, interpretation is said to be on the subjective plane ; it is synthetic or constructive.

All that is most distinctive in Jung's theory of the dream arises out of his doctrine of subjective interpretation ; for it is by subjective interpretation that he finds those unconscious thoughts and feelings whose incorporation in consciousness ensures that fuller adaptation to life which justifies his designation of this method as synthetic or constructive. In dealing with the free associations of the dreamer, subjective interpretation takes account of the feelings and tendencies displayed by the different characters in the dream and regards them as revelations of the unconscious attitudes of the dreamer towards his own problems. Free association commonly leads to thoughts related to the dreamer's sublimations of his infantile tendencies as well as to those tendencies themselves, and in the subjective interpretation of dreams those sublimations which appear in the associative material, but have received no expression in the dreamer's conduct of his life, are taken as indicating the course which he should try to follow in the future. The dream is thus merely a " symbolic " representation of certain unconscious attitudes towards the problem of the moment which are missing from the dreamer's conscious outlook—attitudes or tendencies which he has repressed or neglected. When the associations lead towards infantile sexual tendencies, or even when these are explicit in the manifest content, their occurrence is regarded merely as a means of expression used by the unconscious, and instead of being given concrete value they are interpreted " symbolically " as having a higher, spiritual significance. Thus an incest phantasy in the dream may be held to indicate a need or desire for spiritual " rebirth."

There is a wide divergence between the two schools concerning the nature and interpretation of symbols. The post-Freudians maintain that when the dream is regarded from the teleological or prospective point of view there is no fixed meaning of symbols ; their meaning alters with the psychological situation of the dreamer. They are of the nature of parables—they do not conceal, but they teach. The Freudians, on the other hand, declare that all true symbols have a constant meaning which is not dependent on any individual conditioning factors and always represent unconscious material whose affect is under repression. Much of the discrepancy between the two accounts of symbolism given by the two schools is due to the different senses in which they use th eterm " symbol." The Freudians define it in a very precise way and restrict its use to cases which fit their definition. The post-Freudians use it in a much more general sense as equivalent to " metaphor," or " simile," or indeed any form of indirect representation.

8

Our judgment of the relative importance to be ascribed to these different ways of regarding the dream will depend on what object we have in view in our investigation.   In so far as latent thoughts of the kind found by Maeder, Jung and Silberer are really contents of the dreamer's mind and represent his beliefs, his aims, his hopes, or his aspirations, they are important elements of his personality, and knowledge of them may be useful to him in helping towards that fuller adaptation to life which is the goal of therapeutic analysis.   But although they form part of the latent content out of which the dream is made, they do not seem to have any connexion with the purpose of the dream or to contribute anything towards the forces which give rise to its formation. They are the material which is worked over in the dream-making, but the dream itself is formed by conflict between the repressing forces and the impulses derived from the true Unconscious.

CHAPTER VII

THE NEUROSES

U P to the close of the nineteenth century the great clinical group known as Functional Nervous Disorders occupied a sort of no-man's land between organic diseases of the nervous system and the true insanities. It was made up of two divisions : in one was placed every morbid state that corresponded more or less closely to the classical descriptions of Hysteria, and everything that did not so correspond was relegated to the other under the label Neurasthenia. Sufferers from these disorders did not receive much sympathy or understanding from the medical men of those days and were often made to feel that their disabilities were the outcome of reprehensible weakness and hardly merited the serious attention of scientific men.

These states were classed as Functional Nervous Disorders because they were not the result of any discoverable lesion of the nervous system ; but men trained in the materialistic traditions of the physical and biological sciences found it hard to believe that the mental and physical symptoms of hysteria and neurasthenia were not due to some underlying structural change in the nervous system. Since, however, they were ignorant of the true nature of these states they were necessarily ignorant of how best to deal with them, and a medical student summed up what was known about them at that time when he said that " Functional Nervous Disorders are diseases whose pathology is unknown and whose treatment is *nil*."

During the last thirty or forty years, however, very considerable advance has been made in our knowledge of these disorders and we have now some quite definite notions regarding both their true nature and their treatment. Concurrently with this growth in our knowledge some approach to a scientific classification has been made, and states which on a superficial examination appear to be widely apart are found to fall easily into natural groups in virtue of certain properties which they have in common. All that was formerly called Functional Nervous Disorder is now commonly included under the term Neurosis, and the neuroses are divided into two groups, namely, the Psychoneuroses and the true Neuroses, according as the primary defect lies in the psychical or in the physical domain. Hysteria is a psychoneurosis : it is of mental origin. Neurasthenia is a true neurosis : it is of physical origin. The true insanities are called Psychoses : they may sometimes have a bodily origin, sometimes, probably, a mental origin.

Thus it would seem as if we had not moved far from the earlier classification. It looks as if we had merely re-named the groups marked off by the nineteenth century clinicians. But this is not so. Hysteria is a much wider term than it formerly was and Neurasthenia is a much narrower one ; much that used to be classed under Neurasthenia is now known to be of the same nature as Hysteria.

Janet separated from the neurasthenic lumber-room a great group which he called Psychasthenia—comprising states showing morbid fears, doubts, obsessions, fixed ideas, and compulsions. This group, however, had already been divided by Freud into two, one of which he called Anxiety Hysteria and the other Obsessional or Compulsion Neurosis. Both of these are classed, along with Conversion Hysteria, as Psychoneuroses. As has already been said (Chapter II), the classical form of hysteria is now known as conversion hysteria, because here the painful affect of the repressed wish is converted into physical manifestations. In anxiety hysteria capacity for such conversion is not present and the painful feeling is apprehended as anxiety and dread. This dread occurs in the form of " anxiety attacks " which become associated with certain objects or situations in the external world ; and, as a protective measure for avoiding these attacks, phobias of these objects or situations arise. We thus get two kinds of symptoms in anxiety hysteria, namely, the phobias that serve as a screen behind which the dangerous situation may be avoided, and the " panics " or anxiety attacks that occur if the phobia is disregarded and the feared situation faced. Anxiety attacks may also arise, in the absence of any feared situation, merely from the accumulation of the psychic tension related to the repressed wish.

Another group, detached by Freud from the old class Neurasthenia, under the name of Anxiety Neurosis, includes the greater part of those conditions which are now known as true or actual neuroses. These are so-called because they are regarded as having their origin and causation in the physical, and not, like the psychoneuroses, in the mental sphere. The other two members of this group are Neurasthenia properly so-called and Hypochondria.

Thus according to modern teaching the neuroses comprise two great groups: (1) The true Neuroses, and (2) the Psychoneuroses. The true neuroses are: Anxiety Neurosis, Neurasthenia and Hypochondria. The psychoneuroses are: Conversion Hysteria (with a sub-group; Fixation Hysteria), Anxiety Hysteria and Compulsion Neurosis.

In the preceding pages something has already been said about the psychoneuroses inasmuch as the conceptions of both dissociation and repression, dealt with in Chapters II and III, have arisen out of the study of hysteria. Janet considers all neuroses as being primarily due to a lowering of nervous or psychical tension accompanied by an exhaustion of the higher functions of the brain. Recognizing that some mental functions are easier to accomplish and more resistant to stress than others, he ascribes the difference between the symptoms of psychasthenia and those of hysteria to differences in the level to which the nervous tension has receded. Nervous exhaustion may be brought about in various ways and the consequent lowering of nervous tension leads in some cases to a general lowering of all the mental functions which affects first and most severely those of most recent acquisition.

According to Janet there are two classes of mental operations, one having to do with abstract ideas, memories and imaginations that are not immediately related to our actions; the other, the " function of the real," having to do with the world of present sense-impressions and the reactions by which we seek to modify the world as it appears to us. This latter class of mental operations is more difficult than the former because it is concerned with such a complexity of elements which have constantly to be worked up into new syntheses. It consequently requires a higher level of psychic tension for its proper performance and will be the first to fail if the mental level falls too low. This is what happens in psychasthenia and in this condition there is no very evident restriction of the mental insufficiency to any one localized point. In hysteria, however, probably on account of particular dispositions or of some unknown hereditary peculiarities, instead of a general lowering of function a narrowing of the field of consciousness occurs, and the disabilities resulting from the failure of mental synthesis are more or less strictly localized.

Janet discusses the factors on which the localization of hysterical symptoms may depend and he takes into consideration various circumstances which he thinks may be operative in its production ; but none of these, either singly or in combination, affords a satisfactory explanation of the form the symptoms take in any particular case. The demonstration that the symptom, no matter what its form, has a definite meaning relevant to the personal life-history of the patient we owe to Freud. The possibility of such a demonstration was adumbrated in Janet's earlier work on subconscious ideas, but he has not followed up this line of thought.

Consideration of Janet's views has introduced us to various important conceptions, but his ascription of all psychoneurotic disturbances to mere oscillations of the level of psychic tension proves unsatisfying. His principles fail to account satisfactorily for the occurrence of the psychoneuroses or to give any meaningful explanation of their symptoms ; for the incidence of a psychoneurosis and the particular symptoms manifested therein are ascribed by him to a process which is too purely mechanical and too devoid of any relation to forces within the organism itself.

Freud's theory of the neuroses is inseparably connected with his theory of the *libido* ; and here, as at all times, the precise " sexual " meaning of *libido* in Freud's writings must be kept in mind, in view of the fact that Jung has extended the use of this term so as to make it include every form of interest or striving.   The *libido* related to the production of the psychoneuroses is the *libido* pertaining to those impulses which normally suffer repression in childhood and find adequate outlet in sublimated activities.   Their outlet in psychoneurotic symptoms is one of the possible fates of repressed " wishes " (see Chapter V, p. 89).

According to Freud *libido* is to be regarded as a craving analogous to hunger—a craving which needs and seeks satisfaction from childhood to old age.   In infancy it is distributed amongst the tendencies related to the erotogenic zones and the impulse components of the sexual instinct, as has already been described.   In adult life that part of the *libido* which has escaped repression and sublimation becomes concentrated in the channels which provide satisfaction for the normal love-life ; and if any hindrance to the outflow by these ways occurs there is a damming back of the *libido*, which then tends to regress or flow backwards into earlier channels and to revive those earlier tendencies which are appropriate and permissible in childhood, but are incompatible

with adult standards. The re-animation of infantile
tendencies by such an accession of *libido* leads to a
threatened intrusion of these unconscious " wishes " into
consciousness. This threatened invasion is met by the
resistance of the whole moral and æsthetic nature so
that the admission of these wishes into consciousness
is on no account permitted. Yet the pent-up energy
may be so great that repression partially fails, and the
unconscious desires, not wholly to be gainsaid, break
through in the distorted form of neurotic symptoms,
just as in sleep they break through in the disguise of
the manifest content of the dream. Thus in most
general terms it may be said that every psychoneurosis
results from deprivation of the satisfactions of the normal
love-life and the consequent regression of the *libido* and
re-animation of tendencies to earlier modes of gratification which are unacceptable to the whole personality
of the patient. The deprivation is a relative deprivation
and consists in an inability, for one reason or another,
to apply in an acceptable way the quantity of *libido* at
one's disposal. The result is an increase of psychic
tension, which breaks through the repression and leads
to neurotic illness.

Deprivation may be dependent on circumstances in
the outer world—the many factors which tend towards
unsatisfied love and sexual abstinence in the life of
civilized man. More common, however, and more
important, is the inability to find satisfaction in the
" real " world, rather than in the world of phantasy,
because of inhibitions and conflicts within the mind
itself. Here, owing to infantile fixations of the *libido*,
the individual is unable to give up the satisfactions of
childhood (now being realized in unconscious phantasy)

and to accept the normal satisfactions which life can offer him.

In some cases illness sets in as soon as the irresponsible age of childhood is left behind. This is really an arrest of development, and the individual never attains the plane of normal adult health. There may also occur a relative deprivation owing to an access of *libido*—as at puberty and the climacteric—greater than the individual can maintain in tension, sublimate, or directly apply.

Although this account holds true in a general way of all the neuroses, the particular kind of illness which results from deprivation and regression of the *libido* would seem to depend on the stage of sexual development at which fixation has occurred. Every fixation, whatever its nature, is a vulnerable point in the *libido* development, and it is here that the re-activation of the infantile tendencies caused by regression will be most effective in threatening or overcoming the repressing forces, because of the facility with which the energies roused tend to flow into their old channels of expression. As a rule it may be said that in hysteria the regression is a return to the primary incestuous love-objects involved in the Œdipus complex ; in compulsion neurosis the path of regression leads more particularly to the primitive form of sexual organization—the phase of discrete erotogenic zones and impulse-components not yet subordinated to the genital functions. As we have seen, a narcissistic phase of *libido*-application precedes the phase of true object-love, such as love for the parents, and when regression finds the fixation-point at the narcissistic level the resulting illness may take the form of one of the true insanities such as dementia præcox or melancholia.

The immediate result of deprivation or denial of the normal *libido*-strivings is a turning away from " reality " —an introversion of the *libido* which now seeks in imagination or phantasy the satisfactions which the " real " world has refused. This has ever been the way of human nature when desire is frustrated or when the effort to achieve its fulfilment seems to be beyond one's power. The boy day-dreams of the great things he will do when he grow up ; the limits to his achievements are set only by the limitations of his powers of imagination. So, when a child's actual world is unsatisfying, the pleasurable activities of the past, which he had to renounce in the course of his cultural development, are re-awakened and he lives them over again in phantasy. In doing so he finds happiness in a way to which he ever afterwards tends to return when his longings are thwarted or when he finds life hard.

These phantasies of childhood, like the actualities for which they stand, become subjected to repression and take on an unconscious existence. They lead to no conflict in the mind so long as their intensity is not too great ; but when, through the access of energy brought to them by the backward flow of the *libido*, their intensity becomes so great that they threaten to intrude into consciousness, conflict ensues and some permissible outlet for their pent-up energies must be provided. Such an outlet is found in the neurotic symptom.

Freud's theory of the neuroses which finds their specific causes in the unconscious residues of infantile sexuality has met with opposition and criticism from many sides. But the opinions of only a few of those who have not accepted his conclusions are alone deserving of serious consideration. For the greater part of the opposition has been quite uncritical and based on nothing but prejudice and dislike ; it has been carried on by those who have made no serious attempt to understand Freud's principles or to apply his methods in the investigation or treatment of neurotic disorders ; but there are a few noteworthy instances of men who, though trained in the theory and practice of Psycho-Analysis, have, nevertheless, come to deny the validity of many of Freud's doctrines. In particular, two of Freud's early following,—Jung, of Zürich, and Adler, of Vienna—have deviated in important respects from the teachings of Psycho-Analysis.

Both of these writers repudiate the conclusions of the psycho-analysts regarding the part played by sexuality in the production of the neuroses. Jung minimizes the importance of fixation as a determinant of neurosis and does not ascribe regression solely to deprivation of love and normal sexual satisfaction. By extending the use of the term *libido*, so as to make it include every form of interest and striving, he is able to say that regression of the *libido* results when a person turns back from any task which life may bring to him. It is failure in adaptation to life rather than in true *libido*-satisfaction which, for Jung, forms the starting point of the introversion that leads to neurosis.

In their adaptation to life individuals behave differently, according to the " psychological type " to which they belong. Jung has divided people into four types, according to which of the four psychological functions— thinking, feeling, intuition, and sensation—they habitually use in adjusting themselves to the various circumstances of their lives. In the man whose adaptation is effected by thinking, the feeling function is neglected and sinks into the unconscious, where it tends to remain as a lost capacity, undifferentiated and undeveloped as a function adapted to external situations. Jung admits that the basis of every neurosis is an unconscious conflict, but instead of seeing this conflict as a contest between infantile sexuality and the moral or æsthetic nature, he maintains that "*the neurotic conflict always takes place between the adapted function and the co-function that is undifferentiated, and that lies to a great extent in the unconscious.*" [1]

Thus for Jung the cause of the conflict lies in the present moment and the symptoms represent the un-differentiated co-function, so that in the structure of the neuroses are to be found the elements of his personality, the "values," which are most necessary to the patient for the successful prosecution of his task—his adaptation to life.

Adler's views on the causation of neurotic illness arose out of his studies on organ-inferiority. It is well known that when one organ of the body suffers from any defect the whole system so reacts that compensation for the defect may somehow be effected. According to Adler the whole life energies of the individual who is born with an inferior organ are concentrated on the desire to seek security from the consequences of his organ-inferiority and to find compensation for the feeling of incompleteness which such inferiority engenders. His life is guided by one all-pervading purpose—the desire for superiority and mastery. He sets before himself, in phantasy, a fictitious goal, which is im-possible of realization, and his energies are deflected

[1] *Analytical Psychology*, p. 405.

from the realities of life and spend themselves in pursuit of a feeling of security and a sense of power.

Adler puts this fictitious goal-seeking tendency of the neurotic in the place of the Freudian *libido* and holds the sexual ideas and symbolisms revealed by psycho-analysis to be merely a form of speech through which the " will-to-power " may be expressed. The symptoms are the defences which the neurotic puts up to assure himself against the consequences of his inferiority, to increase his power over his fellows, and to make them subordinate to his will.

In the course of the preceding chapters the nature and source of neurotic symptoms have been indicated in a general way ; but inasmuch as the symptoms and the sources from which they arise differ in detail in the various forms of neurotic illness met with in practice, it may be well to bring together here the salient features of each of the psychoneuroses and actual neuroses as these have been elucidated by the methods and principles of Psycho-analysis.

CONVERSION HYSTERIA

Something has already been said about the symptoms of conversion hysteria. They are the physical manifes-tations seen in the paroxysmal and interparoxysmal phases of the classical descriptions of this disorder. There is no function of the body that may not be impli-cated and the disabilities so produced sometimes simulate very closely those due to grave organic disease. Paralysis and anæsthesia or some over-activity of motor and sensory functions are the most commonly observed defects and may be taken as typical symptoms of this form of neurosis.

A general outline of the development of hysterical symptoms has also been given in the preceding pages. We have seen how, as a result of deprivation and regression of the *libido*, earlier erotic activities of childhood are revived, by way of unconscious phantasies, and come into conflict with the ego-tendencies of the patient. As a result of this conflict a compromise is effected and the repressing forces, as well as the unconscious wish pertaining to the phantasy, achieve some sort of satisfaction in the hysterical symptom which emerges. In the formation of the symptom the same mental processes occur as take part in the making of a dream. Only by condensation and displacement is it possible for the symptom to stand as a substitute for the satisfaction of the opposing wishes. The symptom is not, indeed, recognized by the patient as any form of satisfaction but rather as suffering, and it is through the latter quality that the repressing forces are gratified—the symptom is an expression of the disapproval with which the personality meets the reawakened infantile wishes. But analysis of the symptom shows that it also symbolizes these wishes and provides for the unconscious a substitute gratification of them.

Analysis reveals the infantile experiences out of which the symptoms arise. It was at one time thought that the memories of these experiences were the reproductions of actual happenings in the life of the child ; but it is now recognized that in many instances what is reproduced is only phantasy and has had only psychological reality. The child makes little distinction between fact and fancy, and a similar indifference as to whether a traumatic episode actually happened, or was only a phantasy, seems to govern the production of a neurosis. Whatever is psychologically true, whether or not it be really true, may here be a determining factor.

Among the regularly recurring phantasies revealed in the analysis of hysteria are the witnessing of parental intercourse, seduction by an adult, and the threat of castration. It would seem as if such experiences of childhood, in fact or in phantasy, are necessary for the production of hysteria. But, so far as phantasies of this kind are concerned, there are grounds for believing that they occur consciously or unconsciously in every one; and the recurrence of the same phantasies again and again, in different patients, suggests that these " primal phantasies," as Freud calls them, are a racial inheritance common to all mankind. If this be so it is not the mere occurrence of such phantasies which is important in the production of hysteria, but the fixation or lingering of the *libido* at this stage of sexual development. When through deprivation or denial of its normal satisfactions the *libido* regresses, it first turns towards these phantasies of childhood ; and when the phantasies, reinforced by such access of *libido*, meet with the repressing forces of the personality, the *libido* retreats still further to its points of fixation in the unconscious.

Underlying the psychic mechanisms which lead to this psychoneurosis there is some constitutional peculiarity which determines that it takes the form of conversion hysteria rather than anxiety hysteria. There would seem to be a bodily predisposition in some hysterics which makes conversion of affects into physical manifestations easier than in other people. This predisposition is sometimes more marked in one part of the body than in others and the localization of a conversion symptom may be determined, in some degree, by the special sensitiveness—often associated with diseases or injury—of the affected part. When this happens the resulting condition simulates that which is found in fixation hysteria, but in the latter the bodily sensitiveness plays a larger part in the determination of the symptom and it has a more specific quality. The sensitiveness of any part of the body which becomes the site of conversion in fixation hysteria appears to be of an erotogenous nature, while the sensitiveness in the predisposition to ordinary conversion hysteria has no such specific quality.

ANXIETY HYSTERIA

When the capacity for conversion is not present the end product in the symptom-formation must remain in the mental sphere. It shows itself as morbid anxiety or dread which becomes attached, in the form of a phobia, to some object or situation in the external world. Certain physical symptoms, such as palpitations or tremors, do occur in anxiety hysteria, but these have a different origin and a different significance from those characteristic of conversion hysteria. In the latter these symptoms are the direct outcome of the mental process which they in a sense symbolize, whilst in anxiety attacks they are merely the natural bodily accompaniments of the emotion of fear.

The phobia is the most characteristic mental product of anxiety hysteria. It is, like the symptom of conversion hysteria, a compromise formation. It symbolizes certain unconscious wishes—ultimately, wishes derived from the period of infantile sexuality—and

9

makes manifest the fear with which such wishes would be regarded by the moral self of the patient if they became conscious.   As a means of avoiding knowledge of the existence of such unconscious wishes, the fear which would result from their intrusion into consciousness is projected on to objects or situations in the external world.   These objects or situations come in some way to represent or stand for the repressed wishes, and when they are encountered, no matter how commonplace and harmless they may in themselves appear to be, they serve to arouse in full intensity the fear that would be appropriate and justifiable were the buried desires to become conscious without disguise.   The function of a phobia is to protect the patient from such an attack of fear or anxiety.   It acts as a danger signal and leads to an avoidance of those situations or objects which, because they symbolize or represent the forbidden wish, would cause an attack of acute anxiety or " panic."

Compulsion Neurosis

In compulsion neurosis as in anxiety hysteria the morbid manifestations are confined to the mental sphere. The essential symptom is the felt necessity to act or think or feel in certain ways as if under compulsion by some alien power.   Obsessive acts, ideas and sensations (hallucinations) may be met with, as well as obsessive emotions such as doubts and fears.   The triviality of the actions of the sufferer from compulsion neurosis is often in striking contrast to the urgent need which seems to force him to perform them, but sometimes the impulsion is towards some terrible crime from the mere thought of which he flees in horror, and from the actual execution of which he protects himself by enforced restrictions on his life and conduct.

In contrast to this felt need to perform certain actions he may be thrown into an agony of indecision between two alternative courses of conduct when either of them would be quite appropriate to the occasion and when the choice made is of no real importance. The great significance which the patient attaches to these trivial actions and choices is due to a displacement of affect from processes in his unconscious which are of real significance to him. Like all dissociated processes these are entirely outside his conscious control and hence their compelling force is felt as emanating from some source outside the self.

The symptom in compulsion neurosis is not, as in hysteria, a compromise formation symbolizing the infantile phantasy on the one hand and the repressing forces on the other. It is rather of the nature of a reaction formation ; the compulsion is an over-compensation for the state of doubt which is at the root of the neurosis. In the hysterical symptom the symbolic gratification of the unconscious wish stands out most prominently ; in the compulsion neurosis symptom the repressing tendencies are chiefly emphasized. The conflicting forces do not as a rule become fused in the symptom as they do in hysteria, but manifest separately as compulsions and inhibitions.

ANXIETY NEUROSIS

In all the psychoneuroses the specific cause of the disorder is found in the past mental history of the patient. The symptoms have a mental origin and a definite meaning. In these two respects they differ from the actual neuroses, in all of which the cause is to be found in the present and the individual symptoms have no meaning, i.e. they do not represent or symbolize any mental process or content.

The specific cause of the actual neuroses is to be found in some disproportion between the afferent excitations of the sexual system and the efferent discharge through which sexual tension is relieved. Anxiety neurosis may occur when the sexual life is of such a nature as to permit or lead to undue excitation without normal satisfaction of the impulses aroused. Such may be the case in over-ardent love-making without intercourse, in the imperfect coitus which results from the use of certain contraceptive devices, in the premature sexual experiences to which young persons are sometimes exposed, and in the disproportion between desire and gratification common in middle life. In all such circumstances the afferent excitations are excessive and the efferent discharge is deficient. Sometimes, not only do the excitations not lead on to physical gratification but, owing to mental inhibitions, the normal desires ordinarily accompanying such excitations do not enter consciousness.

The symptoms of anxiety neurosis reproduce all the physical and mental accompaniments of fear and anxiety. In mild attacks there is confusion of thought and embarrassment such as are seen in cases of " stage-fright." In acute attacks the feeling of " panic " or dread may be very intense and is accompanied by the physical manifestations of fear. There may be palpitation and irregularity of the heart's action, trembling of the body and limbs, profuse sweating, pallor of the skin and widely dilated pupils. Nausea, vomiting, diarrhœa, increased secretion of urine, dryness of the mouth and feelings of suffocation may occur.

In the chronic condition which is met with between attacks of panic the signs of acute fear give way to those of a more persistent anxiety. There is a constant feeling of apprehension which becomes attached to one idea after another; but there are no fixed phobias. The occurrence of these in a case of anxiety neurosis indicates that there is present an element of anxiety hysteria.

Such an admixture of anxiety neurosis and anxiety hysteria is indeed most commonly found. Deprivation of sexual satisfaction results from the causes which produce anxiety neurosis, and the deprivation is followed by regression of the *libido* and the reactivation of infantile tendencies as already described. The threatened invasion of consciousness by these tendencies and the conflict that ensues result in their admission into consciousness in the disguise of anxiety hysteria symptoms. In a similar way the presence of anxiety hysteria predisposes to anxiety neurosis : for the internal inhibitions which lead to regression and anxiety hysteria symptom-formation prevent also that adequate efferent discharge of the sexual excitation which alone affords protection from anxiety neurosis. Thus it happens that neither anxiety hysteria nor anxiety neurosis is often met with in a pure form, and, in the treatment of patients both sides of their disabilities have to be dealt with by the methods appropriate to each.

NEURASTHENIA

The condition to which the term neurasthenia is properly restricted is a primary fatigue-neurosis brought about by excessive efferent discharge in the absence of adequate afferent sexual excitations. Excessive masturbation (or pollutions) accompanied by intense moral conflict appears to be the specific cause of this condition. Other factors enter into the production of neurasthenia, such as mental or physical strain and the toxic poisoning of diseases like influenza and typhoid fever ; but in every case of neurasthenia properly so-called the onanistic factor is found, whilst these other factors may or may not be present. It must be borne in mind that this applies only to the small number of cases which constitute the class of true neurasthenia and does not hold good of many of the conditions which are still often grouped under that name. Most of these are cases of anxiety neurosis or compulsion neurosis, the ætiology of which is quite different.

The intensity of the moral struggle against masturbation plays a great part in the production of neurasthenia. When this is present it is always associated with a severe unconscious conflict, related to old perverse or incestuous wishes, which is symbolized in the phantasies that had led up to the onanistic act.

The symptoms of neurasthenia are profound lassitude and exhaustion with inability to concentrate the attention or to perform any continuous work. Complaints of pressure in the head, painful feelings in the joints and muscles, dyspepsia and constipation, commonly form part of the picture. Spinal irritation, diminished potency and general emotional depression are often present.

Hypochondria

The essential feature of hypochondria—undue attention to, and undue solicitude about, the functioning of the internal organs—appears to depend on an abnormal sensitiveness of these organs, so that stimuli emanating from them, which ordinarily attract no attention, become unduly prominent in consciousness. Psycho-analytic investigations point to the probability that this organ-sensitiveness in hypochondria is of an erotogenous nature comparable to that of the erotogenic zones in childhood. Freud believes that these erotogenic areas are not confined to the surface of the body and it would seem as if in those persons who develop hypochondria the internal organs are endowed with an excessive amount of erotogenic power. In them, the *libido*, when regression occurs, flows more readily towards the internal organs than towards the more usual erotogenic zones.

The clear-cut distinctions between the actual neuroses and the psychoneuroses, and between one neurosis and another, which are necessary for descriptive purposes are not met with in practice. Most commonly the conditions we have to deal with are of a mixed nature. Especially suggestive are the connexions which have been discovered between the actual neuroses and the psychoneuroses. A neurasthenic symptom is often the starting-point of a conversion hysteria ; anxiety neurosis often underlies anxiety hysteria ; and hypochondria may sometimes lead on to a true psychosis—dementia præcox.

CHAPTER VIII

PSYCHOTHERAPEUTICS

IN the foregoing pages the importance of psycho-analysis as an instrument of psychological investigation has been emphasized, and the illumination which it has brought into the dark places of the mind and the light which it has thrown on the mechanisms and forces through which the psychoneuroses arise and are maintained, should lead us to expect that it may be found equally valuable as a therapeutic measure. And this is, indeed, the conclusion to which all our experience of mental therapeutics in recent years has brought us. Only when we understand how a psychoneurosis has arisen, and what forces are at work in maintaining it, are we able to understand how it ever gets cured. It is true that cure is often effected by other measures, but our understanding of how such cures are brought about was vague and unsatisfying until it became possible to bring to our aid the insight conferred by knowledge of psycho-analytic doctrines. It is therefore advisable to examine the principles of psychoanalysis as a therapeutic measure before considering other methods which have been in the past, and still are, very widely employed. In doing so we must, to a large extent, reverse the historical order in which knowedge of these matters has come to us.

From what we have learnt about the structure of a psychoneurosis we can readily understand that the aim of treatment should be to bring back to consciousness, in undisguised form, the unconscious wishes which are receiving surrogate satisfaction in the neurotic symptoms, and to induce the patient to find some new solution of the conflicts thus revealed. When this is done the symptoms disappear because the energies which sustained them are withdrawn and find application elsewhere. Moreover the painful feelings related to the repressed wishes become dissipated and lose their intensity, since they are no longer confined to a dissociated part of the mind and thus cut off from other feelings which might have a modifying influence upon them. Further, the unconscious wishes themselves, the whole complex of feelings and desires which underlay the neurosis, are redintegrated in the personal consciousness and subjected to voluntary direction and control. The energies hitherto expended in repression and in the maintenance of the symptoms are now free to be devoted to socially useful ends. This is the goal towards which the analyst sets himself and he alone knows the difficulties encountered before the end is attained. Chief amongst those difficulties are the " resistances "—the obverse side of the repressions—and the overcoming of the resistances becomes the main task of the analyst.

The resistance in analysis is an expression of the patient's unconscious unwillingness to get well—to give up the symptoms which are affording a substitute satisfaction of the repressed wishes. It is also a measure of the strength of the repressing forces and of the pain which admission of the repressed material into consciousness in undisguised form will entail. It shows itself from the very beginning of the analysis in a variety of ways, under various subterfuges, and the analyst's task is to detect it wherever it lies concealed, to bring it into the open, and to induce the patient to overcome it.

On starting the analysis the patient is instructed to note the thoughts that come into his mind and to give expression to them without selection or criticism of any kind. But notwithstanding this injunction repeated again and again, and his promise to adhere to it, he will frequently omit to reveal some passing thought on the ground that it appears to him irrelevant or unimportant. Very often the ideas thus omitted, when given expression to later, are found to be important links in the chain connecting the symptoms with their unconscious sources.

Some patients are so tongue-tied during analysis, yet feel they have so much to say, that they carefully prepare beforehand the topics on which they wish to speak. This appears to be due to eagerness to make the best use of the time during the hour devoted to analysis, but it is really due to resistance and is a provision against the intrusion of unwelcome thoughts. Loyalty to friends, so strong a force in the minds of high-principled people, is invariably seized upon by the resistance for its own purposes, so soon as the incoming thoughts refer to intimate details concerning other people's lives. Especially is this so in regard to the mentioning of people by their names. For a time this may be allowed to pass, but in the end there can be no reservations in analysis ; for, if there are, all the work comes to naught. The resistance will set up a defensive barrier behind which the hidden complexes take shelter as in a sanctuary which may not be violated.

At the beginning of the treatment the patient may be asked to tell all he knows about himself and his illness. If the rule of telling everything that comes into his mind is adhered to by the patient, a consecutive narrative is not to be expected or encouraged. Some patients begin with their earliest recollections and give a history of their lives in which the gaps prove more important than what is told. Others tell the story of their illness and of what they have suffered at the hands of many physicians ; others, again, expand upon some current conflict which is occupying their thoughts. Not infrequently patients begin the analysis by declaring that they have nothing in their minds—that they cannot think of anything to say, and that the analyst should suggest to them what they should speak about or ask them what he wants to know. Such a request is never acceded to, for it is a manifestation of the resistance and must be dealt with as such.

As the analysis proceeds and more and more intimate portions of the patient's life come to be revealed, the personal relation between patient and analyst assumes increasing importance. If the analyst has been tactful and sympathetic the patient soon comes to take up towards him an attitude of trustfulness, accompanied by feelings of respectful regard or affection. This attitude facilitates the analysis and makes easier the relating of intimate experiences and the confession of tendencies considered unworthy. Interest in the analyst soon occupies an inordinate part of the patient's thoughts and is accompanied by an estimation of his character and attainments which is in most cases an overestimation not warranted by the facts.

For a time the analysis may go along well under this

new stimulus, the patient's associations coming freely and their connexions and interpretations being accepted with avidity, but a day comes when a check to this satisfactory state of affairs takes place. The patient can think of nothing to say, or makes no attempt to follow the rule of expressing what is in his mind ; he is apparently obsessed by something which he does not wish to divulge, and it is obvious that some strong resistance is at work. When this resistance is overcome the situation reveals itself as one in which the patient is found to have selected the physician as a suitable object on which to lavish intense feelings of affection (or dislike).

When the analyst is a man and the patient a woman this affection may have every appearance of normal love and is often maintained by the patient to be such, although the circumstances of the treatment and the attitude of the physician have provided no justification for such a development. This situation arises regularly in every successful analysis and, although at one time it was thought that it might be only an unfortunate accidental occurrence which interfered with the thera-peutic work, it is now known to be, not merely an inevitable accompaniment of the analytic process, but the necessary foundation of its successful prosecution. Its explanation is to be found in the neurotic capacity for displacement of affect. The displacement here is known specifically as *transference* ; for the sentiments displayed towards the analyst have not arisen in relation to him and the present situation, but in relation to persons and situations in the patient's past life, or in his life of phantasy, and are transferred to the analyst " ready-made."

The erotic constituent or ground of the love attraction excites strong resistances when it threatens intrusion into consciousness, and the discovery and overcoming of these resistances form an important part of the analytic work. Hostile feeling towards the analyst, as well as a feeling of love, may arise, and here also it is a transference rather than a feeling justified by anything in the actual relations brought about by the analysis. Both the hostile feelings and the erotic side of the feelings of affection are sources of strong resistance ; but on the other hand the conscious, acceptable side of the trans-ference continues to be the most important aid to the analytic work. Indeed, the time comes when the transference becomes the field on which the neurotic conflict has to be fought to a finish, and the transference relation alone can provide the patient with the driving force necessary to solve the problems presented to him when his repressed wishes are restored to consciousness. At this stage the analysis deals, not so much with the revival of forgotten memories, many of which seem indeed beyond recall, but rather with the repetition by the patient, in the transference relation, of all the past emotional situations and impulses, bound up with the origin of the neurosis, which have hitherto been repressed. They do not appear as recollections, but are re-lived during the analysis ; they do not appear as events which have happened in the past, but as an actual relation to the physician in the present.

With the analysis of all the transference relations the conflicts at the root of the neuroses are brought into the open and have to be dealt with so that some satisfactory solution of them may be found. In effecting this the personal influence of the analyst supplies the

motive force which makes it possible. The whole
mental attitude of the patient is transformed in the
overcoming of the resistances during analysis, and it
is only through the power of the transference that this
is obtained. In the end the transference itself is got
rid of and the patient becomes an independent self-
sufficing human being. All the energies of the repressed
libido and of the resistance against it are combined
in the transference, and when the transference is dissolved
the energy is free to become applied to suitable objects
in the " real " world.

Freud says the *libido* thus freed is at the disposal of
the ego, since, owing to the removal of the repressions,
it cannot return to its former objects. Jung maintains, however, that it finds an easier outlet than that
afforded by any object in the outer world : it tends
to sink down into the depths of the unconscious, "reviving
what has been dormant there from immemorial ages." [1]
Thus, he says, is produced a new phase of transference in which phantasies derived from the collective
unconscious are projected on to the analyst just as
the infantile phantasies were ; but the analyst no
longer appears in the guise of father or guardian, or
any other form having a basis in the personal reminiscences of the patient, but acquires the attributes of
god or devil. It is at this point that Jung's therapeutic
methods show their greatest divergence from those of
psycho-analysis. It is no use, he says, attempting to
reduce these phantasies to their component reminiscences,
for these products of the collective unconscious have
no basis in personal experience. He believes that
these images or " symbols " of the collective unconscious

[1] *Analytical Psychology*, p. 411.

have values which are useful for the future direction of the patient's life, but these values are not disclosed unless the phantasies are treated to a synthetic (not analytical) interpretation. The way of escape from the clutches of the collective unconscious is not by way of repression or of assimilation of its contents by consciousness ; its victim can free himself only by presenting these contents visibly to himself as something that is totally different from him. He must learn to differentiate what in himself is ego from what is non-ego, and he is able to do this only if he neglects no part of his duties towards life, but is in every respect a vitally living member of human society.

It is in reference to the task of coming to terms with the collective unconscious that Jung develops his method of subjective (synthetic) interpretation already referred to in connexion with dream symbolism (Chap. VI, p. 112). In theory Jung and his followers admit the importance of reductive analysis, but in practice they seem to lay chief stress on the synthetic or constructive (hermeneutic) method—a method which is fundamentally opposed to the principles of psycho-analysis. In this method the phantasies and dreams of the patient are regarded as containing disguised indications of the lines of development which are most suitable and desirable for him to follow, and Jung declares that " Just as soon as we begin to elaborate the symbolic outlines of the path, the patient must begin to walk thereon. If he delude himself and shirk it, no cure can result. He must really live and work according to what he has seen and recognized as the direction for the time being of his individual life-line, and must continue thereon until a distinct reaction of his unconscious shows him that he is beginning in good faith to go a wrong way." [1]

The psychotherapeutic methods of[Freud and of Jung are regarded, by those who use them, as affording the only radical treatment of the neuroses. But the number of those who adhere to their methods is small in comparison with the number of physicians who use some form of psychotherapy in their practice. Before the methods of analysis were known, other psycho-therapeutic measures were more or less widely used and most of these are still employed by workers in this field. The problem created by the disablement of vast numbers of soldiers in the course of the war, owing to neurotic disorders, led to the hurried training of many men in the principles and practice of psycho-therapeutics, and there is now, in consequence, through-out the world, a much more extensive use of such methods than was possible in pre-war days. Before the war psychotherapeutic practice was confined to a few enthusiasts devoted to some particular method which they had learned from the work of others or had inde-pendently elaborated, but at the present time there are many men who, in consequence of their war training and experience, have specialized in the treatment of neurotic disorders.

The conditions under which treatment had to be undertaken during the war prevented, in the great majority of cases, anything of the nature of a complete psycho-analysis being attempted ; and, fortunately, most of the disorders were readily amenable to other measures ; but a striking concession to psycho-analytic

[1] *Analytical Psychology*, pp. 469, 470.

theory was made by many who did not accept Freud's doctrines and who deprecated psycho-analysis in the treatment of the war neuroses. The principle of "repression," following mental conflict, was widely accepted as the cause of dissociation, and the beneficial effects of "abreaction" of repressed emotion was very widely noted. William Brown [1] in this country and Simmel [2] in Germany have recorded their war experience of Breuer's method of abreaction during hypnosis. Brown used it extensively on recent cases of "shell-shock" with amnesia which he treated in the field hospitals, and the success attained he ascribes to the freeing of "bottled-up" emotion. C. S. Myers,[3] also using hypnosis, secured equally good results by effecting re-association of the dissociated memories without any display of abreaction.

In most of the cases treated, both at home and abroad, some form of mental analysis, combined with the explanation of the nature of the illness, persuasion and re-education, was the plan most widely adopted. Simple suggestion, with or without hypnosis, apart from any attempt at mental analysis, was very soon abandoned by most of those who tried it. The general tendency, however, was to use any method found to be of use in bringing about a speedy recovery—recovery at least to the extent of getting rid of the symptoms and enabling the soldier to return to duty.

Each of the methods used, often in combination,

[1] *Psychology and Psychotherapy*, p. 125.

[2] *Psycho-analysis and the War Neuroses* (The International Psycho-analytic Library), p. 30.

[3] *British Journal of Psychology*, Medical Section, Vol. I, Pt. I, p. 20.

in the treatment of the war neuroses had already been employed before the war in the treatment of the neuroses of civil life. The mental analysis undertaken was generally a superficial application of the principles of psycho-analysis ; the method of abreaction was but a going back to, and an application of, these principles in their earliest phase ; re-education had been already elaborated as a therapeutic method by Janet, Morton Prince and others ; persuasion had been brought to a fine art by Dubois and Déjerine ; and hypnotism and suggestion had a long history reaching back through Liébeault and Braid, to Mesmer and the Animal Magnetists.

In the accounts of the *mental analyses* carried out in the treatment of war neuroses there is an absence of record of the employment of any suitable technique which would make a useful analysis possible. Although frequently referred to as psycho-analysis it is in most cases obvious that the investigation of the patient's mind was not carried out in accordance with the rules laid down by psycho-analysts. These rules are no arbitrary formulations of a particular sect ; they are the outcome of long experience and are adopted as being the best means of bringing to light and overcoming the patient's resistances. And if the resistances are neglected any analysis that is undertaken can only be of a very superficial character. It is not surprising, then, that many of those who claim to have used psycho-analytic methods in the treatment of nervous disorders produced by the conditions of war have remained unconvinced of the truth of the main part of Freud's theory of the neuroses.

The method of *abreaction* is undoubtedly productive

of very striking results in suitable cases; but it is doubtful how much of the amelioration thus secured is due to the discharge of pent-up emotion, and how much to the restoration of lost memories which is at the same time brought about. The latter would seem to be the more important of the two, but the chief factor in recovery is perhaps to be sought in that personal relationship to the physician which, as we shall see, is of paramount importance in every psychotherapeutic method.

The employment of hypnotism for the discovery of dissociated memories and for their *re-association* by means of suggestion was common in hypnotic practice before the war. In many cases of temporary amnesia this appears to be all that is necessary for restoration to health; but the benefit gained for analysis by the broadening of memory during hypnosis was shown by Freud to be illusory if a full analytical investigation is contemplated; for although the resistances are lessened in some directions they are increased in others. The help of hypnosis was, therefore, abandoned long ago in psycho-analysis.

For many years prior to the war *re-education* was, perhaps, the most orthodox form of psychotherapeutics. It was sometimes used to counteract particular morbid symptoms such as hysterical paralysis and other disorders of movement, but it was also applied in more obviously mental conditions. It was attempted by mental exercises to modify mental disorders directly and to educate those mental faculties in which the patient might be lacking. Particular stress was laid on the education of attention, and the value of work for the restoration of intellectual activity was also emphasized.

The consequences of these methods are not always salutary. In neuroses with neurasthenic or fatigue symptoms the efforts demanded from the patient often lead to increased exhaustion and depression. On the other hand education by means of manual or mental work is sometimes of the greatest service. Success depends on accuracy of diagnosis and here, as elsewhere in psychotherapeutic work, good results are in proportion to our knowledge of the mechanism and cause of the malady. In the treatment of the psychoneuroses this implies some form of investigation of the patient's mind, without which we remain in ignorance of the origin of the symptoms and of the emotional experiences related to them. For this purpose Janet relied mainly on hypnosis and other ways of tapping the subconscious ; and when he had thus discovered some of the lost memories connected with the hysterical symptoms, he endeavoured to modify those which he found charged with painful emotion, by substituting for the painful ideas other ideas associated in the patient's mind with memories that were pleasant.

Morton Prince, using similar means of tracing the origin and course of neurotic symptoms, made use of the information so gained to explain to the patient the nature and significance of his illness and to point out to him the changes in his attitudes and points of view that were necessary for restoration to health. In this way he effected a true, if incomplete, re-education of the patient and helped him towards a better adjustment to his life and circumstances.

In thus appealing to the patient's intelligence Morton Prince incorporated in his re-education method that element of rational *persuasion* on which Dubois founded his whole system of treatment. But Dubois abhorred hypnotism and everything connected with it, so that he was debarred from such knowledge as hypnosis may afford of the subconscious factors concerned in the production of neurosis. The futility of appeal to the reason as a means of modifying neurotic manifestations, when the origin and meaning of these symptoms are unknown, is very soon realized by anyone who attempts it. In the phobias of anxiety hysteria, for example, or in the obsessive thoughts of compulsion neurosis, the reason of the patient is, from the beginning, on the side of the physician ; he appreciates as well as does the latter the irrationality of his fears or compulsions, but he is nevertheless powerless against them. The explanation of this is two-fold ; in the first place the root of the trouble is unconscious, and attack upon the conscious phenomena is like trying to put out the fire by pouring water on the smoke ; in the second place the fault is not in the intellectual but in the affective life, and only through the affective life can it be modified or annulled.

The part played by the emotions in the life of neurotics was recognized by Déjerine in his treatment by persuasion, and the consideration he gave to it no doubt helped towards his successful management of these disorders ; but with him, also, the absence of a suitable technique for the investigation of the unconscious militated against the value of the corrective influences which he brought to bear on the conscious aspects of the patient's life.

The good results obtained in the treatment of patients by both Dubois and Déjerine and by others who have adopted their methods are, without doubt, not due to the appeal to the reason on which they lay so much stress, but to that very factor which they most strenuously deprecate and deny, namely, *suggestion*. Babinski, apparently realizing the identity of the psychological process in persuasion and in suggestion, yet looking askance at suggestion as an aid to therapeutics, divides suggestions into two kinds, according to the effects they may produce. All suggestions that are good and reasonable and lead to beneficial results he dignifies by the name of persuasion ; all those that are unreasonable, such as getting a person to believe that it is a fine day when it is actually raining hard, or that have deleterious consequences, such as the production of paralysis in a limb that is perfectly healthy, he calls suggestion.

The persistent depreciation of suggestion which is so commonly met with in the writings of neurologists and others is based partly on an overestimation of the importance of the intellect in the conduct of life, and partly on the well-known connexion between suggestion and hypnotism ; for hypnotism is regarded by many as an " unclean thing." Yet the more we know about psychotherapeutic methods and of the factors on which their successful application depends, the more are we bound to recognize the part played by suggestion in every one of them. It is therefore important to examine in some detail the nature of the psychological process in suggestion, and to trace the growth of our knowledge about its sources and its powers. We may thus be brought to see that just as psychopathology had its beginnings in the despised work of the hypnotists, so the triumphs of modern psychotherapeutics are rooted in that intangible power which Braid and Liébeault demonstrated, many years ago, to an astonished and incredulous world.

Suggestion has been defined by William McDougall [1] as "a process of communication resulting in the acceptance with conviction of the communicated proposition independently of the subject's appreciation of any logically adequate grounds for its acceptance."

The relation between acceptance with conviction of a proposition (belief) and the removal of neurotic symptoms is a problem which may easily carry us out of the realm of psychology into that of metaphysics, and here we must confine ourselves to the empirical observation that in suitable cases a suggestion that a morbid symptom shall disappear is followed by the disappearance of that symptom. This observation is most readily made in cases of conversion hysteria, and the ground of its possibility is without doubt intimately related to that on which the occurrence of conversion depends. Moreover, the induction of hypnosis, as well as effective curative suggestion, is easier in conversion hysteria than in any other morbid state whatsoever. In anxiety hysteria and in compulsion neurosis a hypnotic state, more or less pronounced, may be induced, but it is not as a rule so easy in these conditions to demonstrate the efficacy of suggestion in removing morbid manifestations. When we try to hypnotize persons suffering from the true neuroses, success is still more difficult to attain ; and in the psychoses, such as dementia præcox, paranoia, or melancholia, our efforts almost invariably fail. Along-

---

[1] See *Social Psychology* (14th Ed.), p. 97, and the *Journal of Neurology and Psychopathology*, Vol. I, No. 1, p. 10.

side of this increasing difficulty in bringing about a true hypnotic state as we pass from the psychoneuroses to the psychoses we must put the fact that a very large proportion of people who consider themselves quite normal and who, to all appearance, are free from neurotic disabilities, can be hypnotized without much difficulty. This is perhaps especially true of young persons of either sex between the ages of puberty and maturity ; but the conditions of susceptibility are complex and their respective importance is not easily appraised.

The giving of therapeutic suggestions has not, however, been confined to the hypnotic state. During normal sleep, when *rapport* can be established between the sleeper and the person giving the suggestion—as in the common case of a child who talks in his sleep and is comforted by his mother's voice—effective suggestions can often be given. Further, suggestion has been systematically employed by many psycho-therapeutists in what is somewhat loosely called " the waking state." The customary technique of those who use this method is of such a nature as to make it difficult for the patient to remain in the alert condition which we associate with ordinary waking life. A restful state of relaxation, with closed eyes, is at least sought after and a certain amount of drowsiness is encouraged. The favourite mode of giving suggestions under these circumstances, namely, in a low monotone, is itself a means of inducing a phase of consciousness comparable to light hypnosis ; so that when suggestion is given effectively in this way we may presume that its efficacy is dependent on, or related to, the presence of some degree of artificially induced dissociation. Effective therapeutic or experimental suggestion in what may be considered a true waking state is, in my experience, only possible with persons suffering from hysteria or with persons who have previously been hypnotized. In both of these conditions there is already present a state of dissociation of such a nature and degree as to make easy the acceptance with conviction of a proposition " independently of the subject's appreciation of any logically adequate grounds for its acceptance."

McDougall's definition covers a wider range of phenomena than those included within the sphere of therapeutic suggestion. It covers everything derived from that primitive credulity which is innate in the mind—the tendency to believe everything indiscriminately. Our " acquired scepticism," which leads us to believe in an order of nature, is a result of the contradictions and thwartings of our expectations which ensue when our beliefs are not in accordance with the actual course of things : if we are to live we must believe certain things and not others. In the course of experience a system of knowledge of concrete things is built up and organized within the mind, and propositions that conflict with our organized systems of knowledge are not ordinarily accepted as true unless accompanied by rational grounds of belief. But if knowledge is scanty or poorly organized, the incompatibility of any proposition with beliefs already held may not be appreciated, and in the absence of any grounds for rejecting the proposed idea, primitive credulity comes into play and the proposition is accepted.

Such is the appearance of suggestibility and primitive credulity when looked at solely from the cognitive side. It conforms to the intellectualistic explanation of belief which holds it to be sufficiently accounted for by the bare presentation to the mind of any uncontradicted image. The absence of organized knowledge in the child may thus conduce to suggestibility based on primitive credulity, and the relative dissociation in hypnotic states may have a disintegrating effect on cognitive dispositions already organized, so that primitive credulity may again come into play. But when we examine the circumstances under which suggestion is seen to be actually effective, when we take into consideration the source from which suggestion comes, another factor is found in the affective attitude of the subject of the suggestion towards this source. This factor is derived from the emotional nature of the person to whom the suggestion is given and particularly from the sentiment which has become organized around the idea of the self.

According to McDougall the most important emotions which enter into the structure of the self-regarding sentiment are the affective side of two primary instincts, namely, the instinct of self-assertion or display and the instinct of abasement or submission. The corresponding emotions have been named positive self-feeling or elation and negative self-feeling or subjection. McDougall believes that susceptibility to the influence of suggestion is directly proportionate to the weakness of positive self-feeling and the strength of negative self-feeling, and to the extent to which they are aroused by the relations existing between the person who receives the suggestion and the person who gives it. When this relation tends to excite any sentiment in which the disposition to submission or subjection plays a prominent part, the most important of all the conditions of suggestibility is present.

McDougall's conclusion that the conative force at work in the person accepting a suggestion is commonly the instinct of submission, corresponds, in a general way, with the more specific findings of the psychoanalysts. Ferenczi has pointed out that there is a phase in the normal development of a child which is characterized by an overwhelming desire to believe blindly, to obey without criticism, and to be in subjection to some higher power. This submissive attitude is first adopted towards the parents and is prompted by love, by the desire for affection or by the fear of disapproval. Subjection to the all-powerful father is pleasurable inasmuch as the child identifies himself with his father whose power he himself hopes some day to possess. When this tendency to submission becomes combined with one of the infantile sexual tendencies which are early subject to repression, the tendency to submission is itself repressed and to a large extent sublimated in such forms as religious piety or hero-worship. Suggestibility is, for Ferenczi, the unconscious desire to believe blindly and to obey without criticism which originated in the child-parent relationship, and he holds that in adults, as in children, the motive of this obedience is the wish to be loved. Thus, according to the psycho-analysts, suggestibility is the expression of a latent tendency to be persuaded by love (or intimidated by fear) and is due to the establishment of a relation between the person who receives the suggestion and the person who gives it, which is an unconscious revival and transference of the relation that existed in infancy between the child and a loving mother or a stern and imposing father.

In the technical language of psycho-analysis it may be said that the efficacy of suggestion depends on the presence of *libido*-impulses directed towards the person by whom the suggestion is given. Freud gave the first hint of this interpretation when he expressed the opinion that " the natyre of hypnosis is to be found in the unconscious fixation of the *libido* on the person of the hypnotizer (by means of the masochistic component of the sexual impulse)." [1]

The relation of the " instinct of submission " to the " masochistic component of the sexual impulse " is part of general psycho-analytic theory which cannot be entered upon here ; it must suffice to have pointed out the common basis in " submission " or " subjection " to which investigators, working along such different lines as those of Freud and McDougall, have reduced that susceptibility to suggestion which is so widespread and important in human life, and of so much significance in the Psychology of Medicine.

That a relationship such as that desiderated by the psycho-analysts—a love-relationship, albeit an unconscious one—arises between the hypnotized person and the hypnotist, can hardly be contested by anyone who has had much personal experience of hypnotic practice. In its main features it was recognized and described by Janet, but although its existence cannot easily have been overlooked by other writers on hypnotic suggestion, it is surprising how little its real nature seems to have been appreciated. It was generally

[1] *Three Contributions to the Theory of Sex* (American Trans.), p. 15, Note 14.

described as a *rapport* which is never absent when hypnotic phenomena of any kind are manifested. *Rapport* is not so conspicuous a feature when " waking " suggestion is employed for therapeutic purposes. Here it seems to amount to nothing more than sympathy and understanding between physician and patient. In treatment by persuasion and re-education it is described as the personal influence of the physician, and in psycho-analysis it is openly recognized for what it is and referred to as " the transference." In each and all of these therapeutic relationships it is the same factor which is at work ; it is a *libido*-manifestation which carries with it a curative influence, the amount and permanence of which depend on the way it is used and on the particular feature of the morbid state against which it is directed.

In suggestion without any mental investigation, save such as is implied in the patient's account of his illness, the power of the transference is brought to bear directly on the symptoms ; and its potency is often strikingly exhibited by the almost magical results that are sometimes obtained. But although symptoms may thus be readily got rid of, the underlying mental processes on which they depend are not altered or modified in any way, and, as is so frequently seen, the disappearance of one symptom may be followed by the appearance of a fresh one—sometimes, it is true, one less inimical to health and social usefulness. Indeed, the transference itself must be regarded as a substitute symptom, for into it is poured some of the *libido* which sustains the neurosis and receives surrogate satisfaction through it. So long, then, as the transference exists the patient's well-being is notably augmented, but this is accompanied by an inordinate dependence on the physician which often becomes a burden to him and a source of weakness to the patient. Nevertheless it does often happen, in the treatment of the less severe neuroses by suggestion, that the period of transference forms a bridge which leads from sickness to health. Over this bridge the patient passes from neurosis to life —and life completes the cure.

The mechanism of the cure in treatment by persuasion is, without any doubt, of the same nature. An appeal to the reason as a means of combating the end-products of the mental processes concerned in the production of a psychoneurosis could only have occurred to one who had vastly over-rated the importance of the intellect in the conduct of life, and who had as greatly under-rated the part played by the emotions and the feelings. Moreover, belief in the curative value of persuasion implies a total disregard of the unconscious basis of neurotic disorders.

In re-educative methods, also, the transference indubitably plays a part. But here its power is brought to bear at a point nearer the source of the illness, in so far as mental analysis of some kind is used to discover the unconscious determinants of the symptoms. The pathogenic material, so revealed, may be cleared away and new and better adjustments to life thereby effected ; and in doing this the personal influence of the physician, based on transference, is of preponderating importance, providing, as it does, one of the main sources of the driving power that makes possible the perseverance in effort which all education demands.

It has been customary to assert that suggestion enters not at all into treatment by psycho-analysis. It has rather been insisted that psycho-analysis is at the opposite pole from suggestion and that its results are as different from those of suggestion as are its methods. This is, in a sense, no doubt true ; but it cannot be maintained that suggestion plays *no* part in psycho-analytic treatment or, in other words, that the suggestive power of the transference is not utilized. It has long been recognized that transference is a necessary condition of successful analysis, and Freud himself has pointed out that it is made use of here in the same form as that which it takes in other methods of treatment, namely, suggestion or " personal influence." The difference between its use in psycho-analysis and its use in re-education, persuasion, or " suggestion treatment," lies in its point of application—that is to say, the forces against which its power is directed. It is on this difference that the difference between the results of psycho-analysis and those of other methods of treatment depends.

The power of suggstieon, inherent in the transference, is used in psycho-analysis to enable the patient to overcome the resistances which are preventing him from becoming conscious of his repressed wishes ; and when, the resistances having been overcome, these wishes do enter consciousness, bringing with them the conflicts out of which the symptoms arose, suggestion, the personal influence of the analyst, is needed to help the patient to find new solutions of these conflicts. Here occurs a true re-education—a re-education starting from the point at which the patient's life had originally gone astray. When the transference itself is dissolved, as it is in every completed analysis, its power becomes dissipated and the patient is left free from neurosis and insusceptible to suggestion. This happy result may not always be obtained, but it is the goal towards which all psychotherapeutic endeavour should aspire.

CHAPTER IX

THE PREVENTION OF NEUROTIC ILLNESS

TWO main phases in the history of the Psychology of Medicine have been dealt with in the preceding pages. The first phase culminated in the work of Pierre Janet and gave us the theory of dissociation which proved so illuminating in our earlier studies of the psychoneuroses ; the second phase began when Sigmund Freud formulated the theory of repression. The theory of dissociation helped us to understand what happens to the mind when a neurosis develops ; the theory of repression taught us how it happens and why it happens. Study of the neuroses in pre-analytic days showed us that the symptoms were due to a splitting of the mind and to the uncontrolled functioning of the split-off portion ; but we found no satisfactory explanation of the occurrence of such a disaster and, consequently, we could not learn how to prevent it. Predisposition to neurosis was ascribed to some hereditary weakness or instability of the mind, some innate defect of mental synthesis, which led to inappropriate reactions when any unusual stress was encountered. The psycho-analytic investigation of the neuroses disclosed the important fact that those events in later life which appear to cause neurotic illness have no such power unless they are associated in the patient's mind with previous experiences of a similar kind which have been repressed. By tracing back the origin of the disorder to events or phantasies of childhood and finding there its explanation, psychoanalysis took away much of the importance previously ascribed to hereditary defect as a causal factor in the production of the neuroses, and freed us, to some extent, in regard to them, from the helpless feeling with which we approach the " prevention " of any disease having such a foundation. Nevertheless, in the ultimate analysis, we must recognize some innate constitutional peculiarity, of a general rather than of a specific kind, predisposing to that type of reaction which characterizes the neurotic.

The discovery that the roots of neurosis are to be found in childhood, and that they arise from developmental defects which may perhaps be avoided, has led to the hope that this knowledge can be so applied in the care and management of children that neurotic disorders may be less prevalent in the future than they have been in the past. But the more we know of the complexity of the conditions on which the occurrence of a neurosis depends, the less sanguine are we of being able to prevent its development by avoiding any single one of them. For it is not to be supposed that the sexual factor is the only one concerned in the production of neurosis. It is the specific factor, so far as we can see, in every case ; but in every case also there are adjuvant factors which play their part in the final outcome. The present circumstances in the patient's life which reinforce the internal inhibitions leading to denial or deprivation ; the mental conflicts which accompany such decisions as life demands from him ;

the nature and the magnitude of the "tasks" from which he shrinks; the chances of fate and fortune which lead to undue stress; everything, indeed, outside himself, that tends to make life hard and to withhold from him those satisfactions which his nature demands; —all these play their part in the production of neurosis.

The amelioration of those circumstances incidental to life which are conducive to "nervous breakdown" is a problem which does not find the key to its solution within the domain of the Psychology of Medicine. It is a question of social polity and of cultural and ethical standards to which psychology can but contribute certain important facts for consideration. But the knowledge which psycho-analysis has given us of the ways in which mental development may go wrong is of immediate practical importance for the training and education of the individual life. And, although some of the circumstances operative in the production of neurosis are beyond the scope of any general ameliora-tion of the conditions of life that may be possible, appearing, as they do to the person affected by them, to be the outcome of fate or destiny; nevertheless, in the preparation for life, in the days of childhood and of youth, character may be so built up that when the time of trial comes a man may pass through it serene and undismayed.

The pre-requisite for the formation of such a character is the early acceptance of the "reality principle" and the restriction and the control of the "pleasure prin-ciple" in the conduct of life. The basis of neurotic failure in the future is laid when, in the early years of childhood, there is a lingering at any of those phases of *libido*-development which ought to be abandoned in

conformity to the acceptance of things as they really
are which the growth of the mind demands. We have
seen that the *libido* in regression returns to just those
phases in its life-history in which lingering over infantile
pleasure-giving activities had occurred and an unwillingness to give them up had been shown. In some cases
this unwillingness has reference to the pleasures derived
from the separate impulses which constitute the sexual
nature of the child before these impulses come to be
organized under the dominance of the genital zones ;
in other cases it is related to the pleasures derived from
those early love-objects which had to be given up because
of their " incestuous " character ; in some cases it refers
to those narcissistic pleasures whose persistance is incompatible with the very beginnings of social or group life.

There is one conclusion to which all psycho-analytic
investigation points with unmistakable clearness, namely
the supreme importance of the first four or five years
of life. This truth has been more or less vaguely apprehended from the earliest times and it has been embodied
in many popular sayings and maxims ; but not until
the technique of psycho-analysis was devised did we
have any clear proof of its universal application and
significance. We now realize that the first great task of
the individual life is the management of those infantile
tendencies which are incompatible with adult standards,
and we may reasonably ask if it is within our power
suitably to direct or control this important period of
development in the life of the child. The problems
which have to be solved in childhood are more far-
reaching in their consequences than any of the decisions
of later life. In those few years we pass through, in
epitome, the stupendous transition from the brute to

the human which in history took æons to accomplish. Delicate and precise in the growing child must the process be, and the attempt to guide or control it may well give us pause. But venture we must, for the training and education of the child is part of its inescapable heritage, and we cannot help influencing the growing mind, even if we would. The training of the child during those early years is a task that cannot be undertaken lightly ; the results are far too momentous. It should be our most sacred duty to bring to our aid all the knowledge and insight we can obtain.

Something has already been said of the possible fates of those infantile tendencies whose persistence into adult life constitutes sexual perversion, and we have seen that failure to sublimate them may result in such persistence as perversions, or in reaction-formations against them, leading to exaggerations and eccentricities of conduct, or in a compromise between the tendencies and the repressing forces which shows itself in the guise of neurotic symptoms. The mental hygiene of childhood has as its special concern—a concern which should outweigh all other considerations—the prevention of these untoward fates of the primitive impulses.

The problem of those early years is thus seen to be the repression of the primitive impulses that are distasteful to the ethical and cultural conscience of the community, and the sublimation, or transference into socially acceptable channels, of the energies pertaining to them. As has been already pointed out, we cannot do much directly to assist sublimation ; we can only help to provide suitable opportunities for its occurrence. We are even more helpless in regard to another factor which may be a source of difficulty : the strength of the impulse to be subdued may be inordinate, and beyond our control, except in so far as we may secure that it is not intensified by being encouraged or too lightly tolerated.

If then so little can be done directly to assist sublimation or modify the strength of the impulses, our opportunities for helping the child towards the successful accomplishment of his task would seem to be confined to the modifying of the repressing forces, according to circumstances which may vary with each individual child. When the primitive impulse is exceptionally strong, the repressing forces brought to bear may be inadequate ; but, as a rule, this is not the danger that has to be avoided. The danger rather is that those who have the care of children may make the repression too great and cause it to fall on tendencies which there is no real need to repress. There would seem to be, in many directions, a need to lighten the repressions and to take care that restrictions are not imposed where they are unnecessary. Perhaps the most important error to be avoided is the inculcation of excessive shame concerning any of the bodily organs or functions. The close connexion between the organs of excretion and those of reproduction and between the impulses associated with these functions in childhood and those of normal adult sexual life, leads to an extension of the feeling of shame until everything sexual, even the word itself, comes to be regarded as shameful or disgusting. How widespread is this result of our traditional training needs no demonstration. It is an integral part of the cultural life of our time. And yet, if we can bring ourselves to consider the matter dispassionately, it must seem strange that grown up people should feel abashed at any reference to what lies behind so much of human life.

The evil effects of this attitude are not commonly realized. They are, perhaps, more pronounced in women than in men. Many unhappy marriages, many lonely lives, and many nervous disabilities can be traced directly to this source. For the repressions of childhood are continued into adolescence with unabated force, and the oversensitive shrinking from the facts of life, which is the natural outcome of childhood's training, is reinforced by the conspiracy of silence on these matters which is entered into by those whose duty it should be to guide and to instruct. The victims of this conspiracy often bitterly reproach their parents and educators for having failed to prepare them for what life was to bring. But the parents and educators are the victims of the same tradition ; they themselves suffer from the very repressions which their training tends to perpetuate.

The problem of sexual enlightenment arises in the training of the child as early as the third year. Between the third and fifth or sixth year his normal sexual curiosity, directed first towards the mystery of birth, excites some perturbation and, it may be amusement, in the nursery ; but his earnest questioning receives no satisfaction. His inquiries cause embarrassment in the grown up people who have the care of him, and in whom he has hitherto trusted, and they evade his questions, or, when evasion is no longer possible, they lie to him. Frustrated in his attempt to learn the truth about things as they really are he withdraws into himself, and builds those phantasies of birth which subsequently may play so great a part in his neurosis. As his little life goes on and fresh problems present themselves to his mind he no longer trusts grown up people on topics of this kind ; indeed it is doubtful if he ever again really trusts them in any matter whatsoever.

What then, should parents do when their child's thirst for knowledge turns to these topics ? The rule they should follow is a very simple one, being nothing more than the rule which they themselves—perhaps in consequence of their own duplicity—find it so necessary to impress upon the child, namely, to tell the truth. There is no need, nor is it advisable, to go beyond the question put by the child, but what he is told must be the truth, imparted in such a way as may be suited to his understanding.

The need for enlightenment remains and the dangers of ignorance are no less evident, even when the management of childhood has been so successful that sublimation has been smooth and no neurotic symptoms or excessive reaction formations have developed. There are fresh difficulties and dangers to be encountered in the period of adolescence and in later years. These are best met by knowledge, and youth has a right to know. Those who are old have learnt their lesson, it may be by bitter experience, and they should have a message to deliver to the young. The substance of that message was given by the Preacher, in Sir Henry Newbolt's poem, "Commemoration."

> "O Youth," the Preacher was crying,
>   "deem not thou
> Thy life is thine alone;
> Thou bearest the will of the ages,
>   seeing how
> They built thee bone by bone,
> And within thy blood the Great Age
>   sleeps sepulchred
> Till thou and thine shall roll away the stone.

" Therefore the days are coming when thou shalt burn
with passion whitely hot;
Rest shall be rest no more; thy feet shall spurn
All that thy hand hath got;
And One that is stronger shall gird thee,
and lead thee swiftly
Whither, O Heart of Youth, thou wouldest not."

The second great task of the individual life presents
itself during the period of adolescence. The first
task concerns the fate of the primary impulses which
are incompatible with adult standards. The second
task is the attainment in life of the normal sexual goal
—the bringing of all the components of the love-life
into one harmonious whole which, breaking away from
the phantasy life of childhood, finds satisfaction in a
suitable love-object in the world of " reality."

There is a phase in the child's development in which
he takes himself as his love-object, and finds all his
satisfactions in his own body. But very early his love
fastens on those who minister to his wants and secure
his gratifications. First and most important in this
connexion is the mother. Later both parents play
their part in the growing love-life of the child. The
parents themselves, guided by their own unconscious
wishes, very commonly show preferences in their attitude
towards their children. The father favours the little
girl; the mother idolizes the boy. The unconscious
motive which leads each parent to pour out more love
on the child of the opposite sex is also at work in determining the preferences of the child for the parents.
As a rule, the little boy becomes deeply attached to the
mother, and the little girl to the father. From the
parents they derive satisfaction of their love-impulses,
and the parents remain as the models for their love-

objects for the rest of their lives. And love begets jealousy. The girl becomes jealous of her mother ; the boy regards his father as a rival. These attitudes, it is true, are not often realized in consciousness for what they are, but they form the unconscious ground of much of the irritability and friction between mother and daughter, and between father and son, so common in domestic life.

In the course of time, as the development of their physical natures dimly forecasts to the growing girl or boy the sexual implications of adult love, this threatening accompaniment of their love towards the parents is repressed, and a kind of attachment that would be impossible in the conscious life lives on in the Unconscious.

The love which an adolescent girl is capable of feeling towards some member of the opposite sex is meant by nature to be accompanied by those feelings which we may call the physical side of love. Love directed towards the father would be accompanied by those feelings did they not meet with a barrier in the mind which effectually prevents their appearance in consciousness. This barrier—the incest barrier, as Freud has called it—arose so long ago in the history of the race, and has become in us so strong, that no conception in the realm of sexual relations is so intolerable to us as that of sexual love between parent and child, or between any near blood-relations.

There is therefore little danger that any conscious realization of the natural accompaniment of love should ever enter the daughter's mind in her strong attachment to her father. But the purely filial love which she lavishes on him is often attained at a terrible cost to her own personality. She suffers the great dissociation —the separation of the physical from the psychical side of love—which has marred the lives of so many women. That which should have been one has been split into two. The natural form of her love-life has been mutilated, perhaps beyond repair. Her love for any other man can never be complete. No one ever wholly satisfies her. If she marries she is unhappy. She feels that life holds something she has missed. She is conscious of a want, but what it is she does not know : unconsciously she is always seeking for the father.

The outcome of a too passionate attachment between mother and son may lead to a similar wreckage of a boy's life. So, also, a too great devotion between brother and sister may lead to a failure of both to fulfil their destiny. However beautiful we may consider such devotion to be, we must remember that it is like the pale and delicate beauty of disease and death, rather than that of health and the fulfilment of life. Absorption in the family is a shrinking from the adventure of life ; and to accept the adventure of life should be the privilege and the duty of every human being.

Thus, just as the human task in childhood is to break away from the primitive tendencies which provided the pleasures and satisfactions of our pre-human ancestors, so in adolescence it becomes necessary to break away from the family ties and restrictions which were appropriate to childhood but would prevent the development of free self-determining personality.

Our whole attitude towards the family as an institution and as a factor in social evolution must be reconsidered in the light of psycho-analytic teaching. Much that we have held to be most admirable and praiseworthy is now known to have most baleful results. The loving attachments between father and daughter, or between mother and son, or between brothers and sisters, which we have been accustomed to regard as beautiful and desirable, are now known to hold within them the seeds of mental conflict which may wreck the lives or mar the happiness of these children when they become men and women. Their fate has, it is true, been already largely determined by the experiences of childhood, and by the way their conflicts at that age have been solved ; but the period of adolescence is only second in importance to that of childhood, in that it provides opportunity for loosening or tightening the bonds that may already have been forged.

The great problem of adolescence is to avoid or to undo that unconscious fixation of love upon the parents which prevents or makes difficult the transition to a love-object outside the family. The solution of the problem lies very largely in the hands of the parents. If they have understanding and goodwill they will come to realize that their own selfishness is the main source of their children's danger and the main source of their failure and unhappiness. They must learn that over-demonstrative affection towards their children is a selfish gratification which may lead to that fixation of the child's love which is so hard to undo. The whole future happiness of the child depends on the smoothness and completeness with which at puberty he can break away from the parents and transfer his love to other persons.

And when the children grow up, the parents must be ready and willing to let them go free ; to allow them to break from the family and its attachments ; to encourage them to seek objects for their love in the outside world rather than selfishly to bind them to themselves and the narrow confines of the home. The respect for filial love and obedience, instilled into our minds from our earliest years, is but an echo of the selfishness of those who, when they are growing old, are unwilling to renounce the gratifications of their youth. The craving for love, as for life, is perennial in humanity. It has its roots in the unconscious, and like all unconscious cravings it is selfish. And youth must be protected from the selfishness of those who are growing old. Here lies the justification of the poet when he says :

> " Therefore I summon age
> To grant Youth's heritage."

CHAPTER X

CONCLUSION

THE principles and practice of Medicine have their foundation in the knowledge derived from the study of pathology and therapeutics ; and the specialized branch of Medicine known as Psychiatry, may be said to be based on psychopathology and psychotherapeutics. Pathological changes taking place in the body are the outcome of the same physiological functions and are subject to the same laws as those which are concerned in the maintenance of health. The manifestations of bodily disease are due to a defensive reaction of the organism as a whole against some form of stress which threatens its integrity. And just as pathology may be regarded as a department of physiology, so psychopathology is but a department of psychology. For in psychopathology we study the reactions of the psyche to stress and we regard morbid mental manifestations as being the outcome of a defensive reaction of the mind as a whole against forces which threaten its integrity. And just as in bodily diseases the efforts of the therapeutist are directed towards the removal of the cause of the stress, or to the reinforcement of the defensive forces, so, in disorders of the mind, all psychotherapeutic endeavour is directed towards similar ends. Again, just as pathology may

174

be studied as a branch of physiological science without any consideration being given to the therapeutic implications of its findings, so psychopathology may be pursued as a specialized department of psychology without any regard to the problems that beset the path of the student of psychotherapeutics.

Because of the primary place held by practical motives in the determination of human activity the history of psychotherapeutics goes farther back than does that of psychopathology, and it has seemed to some, in recent years, that there is need to take care lest psychopathology, in its purely theoretical aspect, should encroach too much on the essentially practical domain of the older study. Although it was under the pressure of the practical motive of trying to cure the sick that psychopathology as a science originated, it may be thought that pursuit of the psychology of the abnormal may be followed too exclusively for its own sake without due consideration being paid to the practical utility of the knowledge that may be so acquired. But this is a view the short-sightedness of which has been shown over and over again in the history of science. The disinterested pursuit of scientific truth has been abundantly vindicated by the valuable practical results to which in the end it has so often led.

The desire to base our therapeutic practice on knowledge of the psychological processes underlying the disorder with which we have to deal is but an application in this field of the principles which changed the empiricism of the medical practitioners of some generations ago into the scientific methods of modern Medicine. And just as in the early days of scientific thereapeutics medical practitioners were often compelled, from lack of knowledge or by force of circumstances, to fall back upon empirical methods, so in the field of psychotherapeutics at the present time our theoretical notions have often to give way to the exigencies of practice.

This double aspect of the subject matter of the Psychology of Medicine, according as it is viewed from the standpoint of psychopathology or from that of psychotherapeutics, must be borne in mind when we try to appraise the value of the conclusions arrived at by different workers in this field. To him whose interest is predominantly scientific, whose main object ever is to find the why and the wherefore of things, the practical outcome of any investigation will always seem to be a secondary matter whose consideration may well be left over to some future time. But to those who are daily grappling with the sufferings and disabilities caused by neurotic or psychotic disorders, the question uppermost in their minds may very well be, How does this or that piece of knowledge help us to cure our patients ? It was under the influence of some feeling of this kind that Jung, in defending his contention that dreams should be interpreted constructively as well as reductively, said : " After all for us therapeuts it is a practical and not merely a theoretical necessity that leads us to seek some comprehension of the meaning of the dream. In treating our patients we must for practical reasons endeavour to lay hold of any means that will enable us to train them effectively." [1]

It is no doubt true, as has often been shown in the past, that a method of treatment may be successful in practice although it has no scientific basis that can be discerned. Jung, himself, admits the absence of scientific justifica-

[1] *Analytical Psychology*, p. 309.

tion for regarding the fundamental thoughts and impulses of the unconscious as symbols indicative of a definite line of future development. But this mode of interpretation may have, as he claims, a real value in therapeutics, when the patient is in need of some definite indication of the line which his future development should take. If such a line can be foreseen from examination of the material provided by the patient's unconscious, and if it holds out to him the promise of a fuller and freer life, there is something to be said for a therapy that takes advantage of the indications so provided and uses them as a means of enabling the patient to escape from his neurosis. And, indeed, it is probable that the subjective interpretation of the dreams and phantasies of the patient may point towards just those sublimations of his repressed impulses which are most suitable and effective. If the interpretations are at all justified they will at least indicate a line of development which is more likely to be successful than any that is imposed upon the patient from without. But here lies the uncertainty and the danger of the method. The temptation to impose upon the patient one's own notions of what is good and desirable for him is hard to avoid, and it may be that the indicated line of future development is sometimes a construction of the physician's mind rather than a true interpretation of the patient's unconscious strivings.

It is, however, thought by many people whose opinions are deserving of respectful consideration that the rôle of spiritual director should be openly adopted by the physician in his treatment of neurotic disorders. This view is held by many members of the post-Freudian school and is one of the features in which their practice

12

differs fundamentally from that of the psycho-analysts.
It is a view that is always welcome to the patient,
for, contrary to the effects produced by analysis, it
tends to reinstate the analyst in the position of the
father and to fortify the resistances so that the final
solution of the conflicts may be evaded.   Nevertheless,
in a severe neurosis in which analysis has been incomplete or unsuccessful, it may be the only course left
open, and it may in some degree succeed where analysis
has failed.   From the psycho-analytic point of view it
is a defeat ; it is a return to suggestion—to the personal
influence of the physician used as a means of directly
combating the neurotic symptoms rather than as a
means of overcoming the resistances to self-knowledge
and so securing a solution of the conflicts which are at
the root of the malady.

It may be thought that in the previous pages too much
space has been devoted to the doctrines of psycho-
analysis and that too little attention has been paid to
rival schools of psychopathology and psychotherapeutics.   Moreover, a book purporting to deal with so
extensive a subject as the Psychology of Medicine might
reasonably have been expected to include within its scope
a greater variety of topics and to have provided fuller
information about many cognate subjects of popular
and scientific interest.   In regard to the latter contention, it may be pointed out that the later developments
of the Psychology of Medicine are of so abstruse and
technical a character that it is peculiarly difficult
in any short exposition to render them intelligible ;
yet they are of such surpassing importance, both in
themselves and in their relation to the whole subject,
that any too cursory treatment of them would result

in misrepresentation of the place they at present hold, and of the part they are destined to play, in the Psychology of Medicine.

In so far as it may be thought that the views of the post-Freudian schools of analysis are here inadequately represented, it must be borne in mind that the work of Freud is the foundation on which all subsequent analytical doctrines and methods are based ; and that psychoanalysis differs from some forms of analytical psychology in that it adheres strictly to the principles of science and does not pose as an ethical system or as an esoteric religion.

Not for the first time in its history is Psychology under obligation to the science of Medicine ; but, as has so frequently happened in similar circumstances in the past, academic psychology has been slow in accepting the new facts which have been brought to its notice by the psycho-analysts. These facts, however, have been in the main so well authenticated and have such far-reaching consequences, that they can no longer be disregarded by anyone whose work demands an understanding of human motives. For many years psychologists have been attempting to give an account of human behaviour, but they have hitherto excluded from its purview much that is essential to the success of their endeavour. The insistence on the need for including this neglected territory within the domain of our conceptions of human life and conduct will prove not the least important of the contributions to mental science which have been made by the Psychology of Medicine.

NOTES ON BOOKS FOR FURTHER READING

The topics dealt with in the foregoing pages may, for the purposes of further reading, be classified under five headings : (1) Mesmerism ; (2) Hypnotism ; (3) Dissociation ; (4) Psycho-Analysis ; (5) Post-Freudian Analysis.

(1) MESMERISM

An excellent account of the Mesmeric period is given in Frank Podmore's *Mesmerism and Christian Science* (Methuen & Co.). Detailed reading on this period should not be undertaken by the student until he has become conversant with modern theories on the subject. He may then read with advantage the works of the English Mesmerists, such as Esdaile, Elliotson, Gregory and Colquhoun, and some of the French writings of the period, especially those of Deleuze, Puységur and Bertrand.

(2) HYPNOTISM

The English reader will find an adequate account of this period in Milne Bramwell's *Hypnotism : Its History, Practice and Theory*. A good introduction to the subject will be found in Frederic Myers' *Human Personality*, Chap. V. The works of Albert Moll, Forel, and H. Wingfield and the writings of Gurney in the *Proceedings of the Society for Psychical Research* may also be consulted. The beginnings of modern Hypnotism can be studied in Braid's *Neurypnology, or The Rationale of Nervous Sleep*, and in Liébeault's *La Sommeil provoqué et les états analogues*. Bernheim's *Hypnotisme, suggestion, psychothérapie* is a standard work on the subject.

(3) DISSOCIATION

For an understanding of this phase of theory and practice the works of Pierre Janet should be studied in detail. The English reader will find a good introduction to his views in a course of lectures delivered by him in America and published in English under the title of *The Major Symptoms of Hysteria*. Dr. Morton Prince's writings are also important in this connexion, especially his *Dissociation of a Personality* and *The Unconscious*. The literature of multiple personality is very interesting and instructive. Short accounts of all the earlier records are given in Frederic Myers' *Human Personality*. The most important of the more fully recorded cases of recent years are Morton Prince's account of the Beauchamp case in *The Dissociation of a Personality*, Sidis and Goodhart's account of the Hanna case in *Multiple Personality*, and Dr. Walter F. Prince's excellent record of the case of Doris Fischer in the *Proceedings of the American Society for Psychical Research*, vols. IX and X, 1915–16.

(4) PSYCHO-ANALYSIS

The reader who wishes to gain a thorough knowledge of Psycho-Analysis must study the works of Freud. Many of them have been translated into English. Trustworthy also are the writings of Ernest Jones, Brill, Ferenczi, Abraham, Hitschmann and some others, but much that has been published on this subject is inaccurate and misleading.

The following works of Freud have been translated into English :

Breuer and Freud	*Selected Papers on Hysteria and the Psychoneuroses*
Freud, S. . . .	*The Interpretation of Dreams*
	The Psychopathology of Everyday Life
	Three Contributions to the Theory of Sex
	Wit and Its Relation to the Unconscious
	Delusion and Dream
	Totem and Taboo
	The History of the Psycho-analytic Movement
	A General Introduction to Psycho-Analysis.

(The last-named work is an American translation of twenty-eight lectures delivered to laymen. An English translation is announced (Allen & Unwin)).

There are also translations of the following :

Ferenczi . . .	*Contributions to Psycho-Analysis*
Pfister	*The Psycho-analytic Method*
Abraham . . .	*Dreams and Myths*
Hitschmann . .	Freud's *Theory of the Neuroses*.

Apart from translations the most important works on Psycho-Analysis in English are :

Ernest Jones . . *Papers on Psycho-Analysis*
Treatment of the Neuroses
Frink . . . . *Morbid Fears and Compulsions*
Brill . . . . *Psychanalysis : Its Theory and Practical Application*
Putnam : . . . *Addresses on Psycho-Analysis.*

(5) POST-FREUDIAN ANALYSIS

The work of the Post-Freudian School may be studied in the writings of Jung, Silberer, Maeder and Adler. The following have been translated into English :

C. G. Jung . . *Studies in Word-Association*
Analytical Psychology
Psychology of the Unconscious.

(A translation of Jung's latest work on Psychological Types is in preparation.)

H. Silberer . . *Problems of Mysticism and its Symbolism*
A. E. Maeder . *The Dream Problem*
A. Adler . . . *Organ Inferiority and its Psychical Compensation*
The Neurotic Constitution.

INDEX

Printed in Great Britain
by BUTLER & TANNER,
Frome and London

A SELECTION FROM

MESSRS. METHUEN'S PUBLICATIONS

This Catalogue contains only a selection of the more important books published by Messrs. Methuen. A complete catalogue of their publications may be obtained on application.

Bain (F. W.)—
A DIGIT OF THE MOON: A Hindoo Love Story. THE DESCENT OF THE SUN: A Cycle of Birth. A HEIFER OF THE DAWN. IN THE GREAT GOD'S HAIR. A DRAUGHT OF THE BLUE. AN ESSENCE OF THE DUSK. AN INCARNATION OF THE SNOW. A MINE OF FAULTS. THE ASHES OF A GOD. BUBBLES OF THE FOAM. A SYRUP OF THE BEES. THE LIVERY OF EVE. THE SUBSTANCE OF A DREAM. *All Fcap. 8vo. 5s. net.* AN ECHO OF THE SPHERES. *Wide Demy. 12s. 6d. net.*

Balfour (Graham). THE LIFE OF ROBERT LOUIS STEVENSON. *Fifteenth Edition. In one Volume. Cr. 8vo. Buckram. 7s. 6d. net.*

Belloc (H.)—
PARIS, 8s. 6d. net. HILLS AND THE SEA, 6s. net. ON NOTHING AND KINDRED SUBJECTS, 6s. net. ON EVERYTHING, 6s. net. ON SOMETHING, 6s. net. FIRST AND LAST, 6s. net. THIS AND THAT AND THE OTHER, 6s. net. MARIE ANTOINETTE, 18s. net. THE PYRENEES, 10s. 6d. net.

Bloemfontein (Bishop of). ARA CŒLI: AN ESSAY IN MYSTICAL THEOLOGY. *Seventh Edition. Cr. 8vo. 5s. net.*
FAITH AND EXPERIENCE. *Third Edition. Cr. 8vo. 5s. net.*
THE CULT OF THE PASSING MOMENT. *Fourth Edition. Cr. 8vo. 5s. net.*
THE ENGLISH CHURCH AND REUNION. *Cr. 8vo. 5s. net.*
SCALA MUNDI. *Cr. 8vo. 4s. 6d net.*

Chesterton (G. K.)—
THE BALLAD OF THE WHITE HORSE. ALL THINGS CONSIDERED. TREMENDOUS TRIFLES. ALARMS AND DISCURSIONS. A MISCELLANY OF MEN. *All Fcap. 8vo. 6s. net.* WINE, WATER, AND SONG. *Fcap. 8vo. 1s. 6d. net.* THE USES OF DIVERSITY. 6s. net.

Clutton-Brock (A.). WHAT IS THE KINGDOM OF HEAVEN? *Fourth Edition. Fcap. 8vo. 5s. net.*
ESSAYS ON ART. *Second Edition. Fcap. 8vo. 5s. net.*
ESSAYS ON BOOKS. *Fcap. 8vo. 6s. net.*
MORE ESSAYS ON BOOKS. *Fcap. 8vo. 6s. net.*

Cole (G. D. H.). SOCIAL THEORY. *Cr. 8vo. 5s. net.*

Conrad (Joseph). THE MIRROR OF THE SEA: Memories and Impressions. *Fourth Edition. Fcap. 8vo. 6s. net.*

Einstein (A.). RELATIVITY: THE SPECIAL AND THE GENERAL THEORY. Translated by ROBERT W. LAWSON. *Third Edition. Cr. 8vo. 5s. net.*

Eliot (T. S.). THE SACRED WOOD: ESSAYS ON POETRY. *Fcap. 8vo. 6s. net.*

Fyleman (Rose.). FAIRIES AND CHIMNEYS. *Fcap. 8vo. Eighth Edition. 3s. 6d. net.*
THE FAIRY GREEN. *Third Edition. Fcap. 8vo. 3s. 6d. net.*

Gibbins (H. de B.). INDUSTRY IN ENGLAND: HISTORICAL OUTLINES. With Maps and Plans. *Tenth Edition. Demy 8vo. 12s. 6d. net.*
THE INDUSTRIAL HISTORY OF ENGLAND. With 5 Maps and a Plan. *Twenty-seventh Edition. Cr. 8vo. 5s.*

Gibbon (Edward). THE DECLINE AND FALL OF THE ROMAN EMPIRE. Edited, with Notes, Appendices, and Maps, by J. B. BURY. Illustrated. *Each 12s. 6d. net.* Also in *Seven Volumes. Cr. 8vo. Each 7s. net.*

Glover (T. R.). THE CONFLICT OF RELIGIONS IN THE EARLY ROMAN EMPIRE. *Ninth Edition. Demy 8vo. 10s. 6d. net.*
POETS AND PURITANS. *Second Edition. Demy 8vo. 10s. 6d. net.*
FROM PERICLES TO PHILIP. *Third Edition. Demy 8vo. 10s. 6d. net.*
VIRGIL. *Fourth Edition. Demy 8vo. 10s. 6d. net.*
THE CHRISTIAN TRADITION AND ITS VERIFICATION. (The Angus Lecture for 1912.) *Second Edition. Cr. 8vo. 6s. net.*

Grahame (Kenneth). THE WIND IN THE WILLOWS. *Eleventh Edition. Cr. 8vo. 7s. 6d. net.*

Hall (H. R.). THE ANCIENT HISTORY OF THE NEAR EAST FROM THE EARLIEST TIMES TO THE BATTLE OF SALAMIS. Illustrated. *Fifth Edition. Demy 8vo. 21s. net.*

Hawthorne (Nathaniel). THE SCARLET LETTER. With 31 Illustrations in Colour by HUGH THOMSON. *Wide Royal 8vo. 31s. 6d. net.*

Holdsworth (W. S.). A HISTORY OF ENGLISH LAW. *Vols. I., II., III. Each Second Edition. Demy 8vo. Each* 15s. *net.*

Inge (W. R.). CHRISTIAN MYSTICISM. (The Bampton Lectures of 1899.) *Fourth Edition. Cr. 8vo.* 7s. 6d. *net.*

Jenks (E.). AN OUTLINE OF ENGLISH LOCAL GOVERNMENT. *Fourth Edition.* Revised by R. C. K. ENSOR. *Cr. 8vo.* 5s. *net.*

A SHORT HISTORY OF ENGLISH LAW: FROM THE EARLIEST TIMES TO THE END OF THE YEAR 1911. *Second Edition, revised. Demy 8vo.* 12s. 6d. *net.*

Julian (Lady) of Norwich. REVELATIONS OF DIVINE LOVE. Edited by GRACE WARRACK. *Seventh Edition. Cr. 8vo.* 5s. *net.*

Keats (John). POEMS. Edited, with Introduction and Notes, by E. DE SÉLINCOURT. With a Frontispiece in Photogravure. *Fourth Edition. Demy 8vo.* 12s. 6d. *net.*

Kidd (Benjamin). THE SCIENCE OF POWER. *Ninth Edition. Crown 8vo.* 7s. 6d. *net.*

SOCIAL EVOLUTION. *Demy 8vo.* 8s. 6d. *net.*

Kipling (Rudyard). BARRACK-ROOM BALLADS. 208th *Thousand. Cr. 8vo. Buckram,* 7s. 6d. *net. Also Fcap. 8vo. Cloth,* 6s. *net; leather,* 7s. 6d. *net.* Also a Service Edition. *Two Volumes. Square fcap. 8vo. Each* 3s. *net.*

THE SEVEN SEAS. 157th *Thousand. Cr. 8vo. Buckram,* 7s. 6d. *net. Also Fcap. 8vo. Cloth,* 6s. *net; leather,* 7s. 6d. *net.* Also a Service Edition. *Two Volumes. Square fcap. 8vo. Each* 3s. *net.*

THE FIVE NATIONS. 126th *Thousand. Cr. 8vo. Buckram,* 7s. 6d. *net. Also Fcap. 8vo. Cloth,* 6s. *net; leather,* 7s. 6d. *net.* Also a Service Edition. *Two Volumes. Square fcap. 8vo. Each* 3s. *net.*

DEPARTMENTAL DITTIES. 94th *Thousand. Cr. 8vo. Buckram,* 7s. 6d. *net. Also Fcap. 8vo. Cloth,* 6s. *net; leather,* 7s. 6d. *net.* Also a Service Edition. *Two Volumes. Square fcap. 8vo. Each* 3s. *net.*

THE YEARS BETWEEN. *Cr. 8vo. Buckram,* 7s. 6d. *net. Also on thin paper. Fcap. 8vo. Blue cloth,* 6s. *net; Limp lambskin,* 7s. 6d. *net.* Also a Service Edition. *Two Volumes. Square fcap. 8vo. Each* 3s. *net.*

HYMN BEFORE ACTION. Illuminated. *Fcap. 4to.* 1s. 6d. *net.*

RECESSIONAL. Illuminated. *Fcap. 4to.* 1s. 6d. *net.*

TWENTY POEMS FROM RUDYARD KIPLING. 360th *Thousand. Fcap. 8vo.* 1s. *net.*

Lamb (Charles and Mary). THE COMPLETE WORKS. Edited by E. V. LUCAS. *A New and Revised Edition in Six Volumes. With Frontispieces. Fcap. 8vo. Each* 6s. *net.* The volumes are :—
I. MISCELLANEOUS PROSE. II. ELIA AND THE LAST ESSAY OF ELIA. III. BOOKS FOR CHILDREN. IV. PLAYS AND POEMS V. and VI. LETTERS.

THE ESSAYS OF ELIA. With an Introduction by E. V. LUCAS, and 28 Illustrations by A. GARTH JONES. *Fcap. 8vo.* 5s. *net.*

Lankester (Sir Ray). SCIENCE FROM AN EASY CHAIR. Illustrated. *Thirteenth Edition. Cr. 8vo.* 7s. 6d. *net.*

MORE SCIENCE FROM AN EASY CHAIR. Illustrated. *Third Edition. Cr. 8vo.* 7s. 6d. *net.*

DIVERSIONS OF A NATURALIST. Illustrated. *Third Edition. Cr. 8vo.* 7s. 6d. *net.*

SECRETS OF EARTH AND SEA. *Cr. 8vo.* 8s. 6d. *net.*

Lodge (Sir Oliver). MAN AND THE UNIVERSE: A STUDY OF THE INFLUENCE OF THE ADVANCE IN SCIENTIFIC KNOWLEDGE UPON OUR UNDERSTANDING OF CHRISTIANITY. *Ninth Edition. Crown 8vo.* 7s. 6d. *net.*

THE SURVIVAL OF MAN: A STUDY IN UNRECOGNISED HUMAN FACULTY. *Seventh Edition. Cr. 8vo.* 7s. 6d. *net.*

MODERN PROBLEMS. *Cr. 8vo.* 7s. 6d. *net.*

RAYMOND; OR LIFE AND DEATH. Illustrated. *Twelfth Edition. Demy 8vo.* 15s. *net.*

Lucas (E. V.).
THE LIFE OF CHARLES LAMB, 2 *vols.,* 21s. *net.* A WANDERER IN HOLLAND, 10s. 6d. *net.* A WANDERER IN LONDON, 10s. *net.* LONDON REVISITED, 10s. 6d. *net.* A WANDERER IN PARIS, 10s. 6d. *net* and 6s. *net.* A WANDERER IN FLORENCE, 10s. 6d. *net.* A WANDERER IN VENICE, 10s. 6d. *net.* THE OPEN ROAD: A Little Book for Wayfarers, 6s. 6d. *net* and 7s. 6d. *net.* THE FRIENDLY TOWN: A Little Book for the Urbane, 6s. *net.* FIRESIDE AND SUNSHINE, 6s. *net.* CHARACTER AND COMEDY, 6s. *net.* THE GENTLEST ART: A Choice of Letters by Entertaining Hands, 6s. 6d. *net.* THE SECOND POST, 6s. *net.* HER INFINITE VARIETY: A Feminine Portrait Gallery, 6s. *net.* GOOD COMPANY: A Rally of Men, 6s. *net.* ONE DAY AND ANOTHER, 6s. *net.* OLD LAMPS FOR NEW, 6s. *net.* LOITERER'S HARVEST, 6s. *net.* CLOUD AND SILVER, 6s. *net.* A BOSWELL OF BAGHDAD, AND OTHER ESSAYS, 6s. *net.* 'TWIXT EAGLE AND DOVE, 6s. *net.* THE PHANTOM JOURNAL, AND OTHER ESSAYS AND DIVERSIONS, 6s. *net.* SPECIALLY SELECTED: A Choice of Essays. 7s. 6d. *net.* THE BRITISH SCHOOL: An Anecdotal Guide to the British Painters and Paintings in the National Gallery, 6s. *net.* TRAVEL NOTES.

McDougall (William). AN INTRODUC-TION TO SOCIAL PSYCHOLOGY. *Sixteenth Edition. Cr. 8vo. 8s. net.*
BODY AND MIND: A HISTORY AND A DEFENCE OF ANIMISM. *Fifth Edition. Demy 8vo. 12s. 6d. net.*

Maeterlinck (Maurice)—
THE BLUE BIRD: A Fairy Play in Six Acts, *6s. net.* MARY MAGDALENE; A Play in Three Acts, *5s. net.* DEATH, *3s. 6d. net.* OUR ETERNITY, *6s. net.* THE UNKNOWN GUEST, *6s. net.* POEMS, *5s. net.* THE WRACK OF THE STORM, *6s. net.* THE MIRACLE OF ST. ANTHONY: A Play in One Act, *3s. 6d. net.* THE BURGOMASTER OF STILEMONDE: A Play in Three Acts, *5s. net.* THE BETROTHAL; or, The Blue Bird Chooses, *6s. net.* MOUNTAIN PATHS, *6s. net.* THE STORY OF TYLTYL, *21s. net.*

Milne (A. A.). THE DAY'S PLAY. THE HOLIDAY ROUND. ONCE A WEEK. *All Cr. 8vo. 7s. net.* NOT THAT IT MATTERS. *Fcap. 8vo. 6s. net.* IF I MAY. *Fcap. 8vo. 6s. net.*

Oxenham (John)—
BEES IN AMBER; A Little Book of Thought-ful Verse. ALL'S WELL: A Collection of War Poems. THE KING'S HIGH WAY. THE VISION SPLENDID. THE FIERY CROSS. HIGH ALTARS: The Record of a Visit to the Battlefields of France and Flanders. HEARTS COURAGEOUS. ALL CLEAR! WINDS OF THE DAWN. *All Small Pott 8vo. Paper, 1s. 3d. net; cloth boards, 2s. net.* GENTLEMEN—THE KING, *2s. net.*

Petrie (W. M. Flinders). A HISTORY OF EGYPT. Illustrated. *Six Volumes. Cr. 8vo. Each 9s. net.*
VOL. I. FROM THE 1ST TO THE XVITH DYNASTY. *Ninth Edition. (10s. 6d. net.)*
VOL. II. THE XVIITH AND XVIIITH DYNASTIES. *Sixth Edition.*
VOL. III. XIXTH TO XXXTH DYNASTIES. *Second Edition.*
VOL. IV. EGYPT UNDER THE PTOLEMAIC DYNASTY. J. P. MAHAFFY. *Second Edition.*
VOL. V. EGYPT UNDER ROMAN RULE. J. G. MILNE. *Second Edition.*
VOL. VI. EGYPT IN THE MIDDLE AGES. STANLEY LANE POOLE. *Second Edition.*
SYRIA AND EGYPT, FROM THE TELL EL AMARNA LETTERS. *Cr. 8vo. 5s. net.*
EGYPTIAN TALES. Translated from the Papyri. First Series, IVth to XIIth Dynasty. Illustrated. *Third Edition. Cr. 8vo. 5s. net.*
EGYPTIAN TALES. Translated from the Papyri. Second Series, XVIIITH to XIXTH Dynasty. Illustrated. *Second Edition. Cr. 8vo. 5s. net.*

Pollard (A. F.). A SHORT HISTORY OF THE GREAT WAR. With 19 Maps. *Second Edition. Cr. 8vo. 10s. 6d. net.*

Price (L. L.). A SHORT HISTORY OF POLITICAL ECONOMY IN ENGLAND FROM ADAM SMITH TO ARNOLD TOYNBEE. *Tenth Edition. Cr. 8vo. 5s. net.*

Reid (G. Archdall). THE LAWS OF HEREDITY. *Second Edition. Demy 8vo. £1 1s. net.*

Robertson (C. Grant). SELECT STAT-UTES, CASES, AND DOCUMENTS, 1660–1832. *Third Edition. Demy 8vo. 15s. net.*

Selous (Edmund). TOMMY SMITH'S ANIMALS. Illustrated. *Nineteenth Edi-tion. Fcap. 8vo. 3s. 6d. net.*
TOMMY SMITH'S OTHER ANIMALS. Illustrated. *Eleventh Edition. Fcap. 8vo. 3s. 6d. net.*
TOMMY SMITH AT THE ZOO. Illus-trated. *Fourth Edition. Fcap. 8vo. 2s. 9d.*
TOMMY SMITH AGAIN AT THE ZOO. Illustrated. *Second Edition. Fcap. 8vo. 2s. 9d.*
JACK'S INSECTS. *Popular Edition. Cr. 8vo. 3s. 6d.*
JACK'S OTHER INSECTS. *Cr. 8vo. 3s. 6d.*

Shelley (Percy Bysshe). POEMS. With an Introduction by A. CLUTTON-BROCK and Notes by C. D. LOCOCK. *Two Volumes. Demy 8vo. £1 1s. net.*

Smith (Adam). THE WEALTH OF NATIONS. Edited by EDWIN CANNAN. *Two Volumes. Second Edition. Demy 8vo. £1 10s. net.*

Stevenson (R. L.). THE LETTERS OF ROBERT LOUIS STEVENSON. Edited by Sir SIDNEY COLVIN. *A New Re-arranged Edition in four volumes. Fourth Edition. Fcap. 8vo. Each 6s. net.*

Surtees (R. S.). HANDLEY CROSS. Illustrated. *Ninth Edition. Fcap. 8vo. 7s. 6d. net.*
MR. SPONGE'S SPORTING TOUR. Illustrated. *Fifth Edition. Fcap. 8vo. 7s. 6d. net.*
ASK MAMMA: OR, THE RICHEST COMMONER IN ENGLAND. Illus-trated. *Second Edition. Fcap. 8vo. 7s. 6d. net.*
JORROCKS'S JAUNTS AND JOLLI-TIES. Illustrated. *Seventh Edition. Fcap. 8vo. 6s. net.*
MR. FACEY ROMFORD'S HOUNDS. Illustrated. *Fourth Edition. Fcap. 8vo. 7s. 6d. net.*
HAWBUCK GRANGE; OR, THE SPORT-ING ADVENTURES OF THOMAS SCOTT, ESQ. Illustrated. *Fcap. 8vo. 6s. net.*
PLAIN OR RINGLETS? Illustrated. *Fcap. 8vo. 7s. 6d. net.*
HILLINGDON HALL. With 12 Coloured Plates by WILDRAKE, HEATH, and JELLI-COE. *Fcap. 8vo. 7s. 6d. net.*

Tilden (W. T.). THE ART OF LAWN TENNIS. Illustrated. *Cr. 8vo. 6s. net.*

Tileston (Mary W.). DAILY STRENGTH FOR DAILY NEEDS. *Twenty-seventh Edition. Medium 16mo. 3s. 6d. net.*

Underhill (Evelyn). MYSTICISM. A Study in the Nature and Development of Man's Spiritual Consciousness. *Eighth Edition. Demy 8vo. 15s. net.*

Vardon (Harry). HOW TO PLAY GOLF. Illustrated. *Thirteenth Edition. Cr. 8vo. 5s. net.*

Waterhouse (Elizabeth). A LITTLE BOOK OF LIFE AND DEATH. *Twentieth Edition. Small Pott 8vo. Cloth, 2s. 6d. net.*

Wells (J.). A SHORT HISTORY OF ROME. *Seventeenth Edition.* With 3 Maps. *Cr. 8vo. 6s.*

Wilde (Oscar). THE WORKS OF OSCAR WILDE. *Fcap. 8vo. Each 6s. 6d. net.*
I. LORD ARTHUR SAVILE'S CRIME AND THE PORTRAIT OF MR. W. H. II. THE DUCHESS OF PADUA. III. POEMS. IV. LADY WINDERMERE'S FAN. V. A WOMAN OF NO IMPORTANCE. VI. AN IDEAL HUSBAND. VII. THE IMPORTANCE OF BEING EARNEST. VIII. A HOUSE OF POMEGRANATES. IX. INTENTIONS. X. DE PROFUNDIS AND PRISON LETTERS. XI. ESSAYS. XII. SALOMÉ, A FLORENTINE TRAGEDY, and LA SAINTE COURTISANE. XIII. A CRITIC IN PALL MALL. XIV. SELECTED PROSE OF OSCAR WILDE. XV. ART AND DECORATION.
A HOUSE OF POMEGRANATES. Illustrated. *Cr. 4to. 21s. net.*

Yeats (W. B.). A BOOK OF IRISH VERSE. *Fourth Edition. Cr. 8vo. 7s. net.*

PART II.—A SELECTION OF SERIES

Ancient Cities

General Editor, SIR B. C. A. WINDLE

Cr. 8vo. 6s. net each volume

With Illustrations by E. H. NEW, and other Artists

BRISTOL. CANTERBURY. CHESTER. DUBLIN. | EDINBURGH. LINCOLN. SHREWSBURY. WELLS and GLASTONBURY.

The Antiquary's Books

General Editor, J. CHARLES COX

Demy 8vo. 10s. 6d. net each volume

With Numerous Illustrations

ANCIENT PAINTED GLASS IN ENGLAND. ARCHÆOLOGY AND FALSE ANTIQUITIES. THE BELLS OF ENGLAND. THE BRASSES OF ENGLAND. THE CASTLES AND WALLED TOWNS OF ENGLAND. CELTIC ART IN PAGAN AND CHRISTIAN TIMES. CHURCHWARDENS' ACCOUNTS. THE DOMESDAY INQUEST. ENGLISH CHURCH FURNITURE. ENGLISH COSTUME. ENGLISH MONASTIC LIFE. ENGLISH SEALS. FOLK-LORE AS AN HISTORICAL SCIENCE. THE GILDS AND COMPANIES OF LONDON. THE HERMITS AND ANCHORITES OF ENGLAND. THE MANOR AND MANORIAL RECORDS. THE MEDIÆVAL HOSPITALS OF ENGLAND. OLD ENGLISH INSTRUMENTS OF MUSIC. OLD ENGLISH LIBRARIES. OLD SERVICE BOOKS OF THE ENGLISH CHURCH. PARISH LIFE IN MEDIÆVAL ENGLAND. THE PARISH REGISTERS OF ENGLAND. REMAINS OF THE PREHISTORIC AGE IN ENGLAND. THE ROMAN ERA IN BRITAIN. ROMANO-BRITISH BUILDINGS AND EARTHWORKS. THE ROYAL FORESTS OF ENGLAND. THE SCHOOLS OF MEDIEVAL ENGLAND. SHRINES OF BRITISH SAINTS.

The Arden Shakespeare

General Editor, R. H. CASE

Demy 8vo. 6s. net each volume

An edition of Shakespeare in Single Plays; each edited with a full Introduction, Textual Notes, and a Commentary at the foot of the page.

Classics of Art

Edited by Dr. J. H. W. LAING

With numerous Illustrations. Wide Royal 8vo

THE ART OF THE GREEKS, 15s. net. THE ART OF THE ROMANS, 16s. net. CHARDIN, 15s. net. DONATELLO, 16s. net. GEORGE ROMNEY, 15s. net. GHIRLANDAIO, 15s. net. LAWRENCE, 25s. net. MICHELANGELO, 15s. net. RAPHAEL, 15s. net. REMBRANDT'S ETCHINGS, Two Vols., 25s. net. TINTORETTO, 16s. net. TITIAN, 16s. net. TURNER'S SKETCHES AND DRAWINGS, 15s. net. VELAZQUEZ, 15s. net.

The 'Complete' Series

Fully Illustrated. Demy 8vo

THE COMPLETE AMATEUR BOXER, 10s. 6d. net. THE COMPLETE ASSOCIATION FOOTBALLER, 10s. 6d. net. THE COMPLETE ATHLETIC TRAINER, 10s. 6d. net. THE COMPLETE BILLIARD PLAYER, 12s. 6d. net. THE COMPLETE COOK, 10s. 6d. net. THE COMPLETE CRICKETER, 10s. 6d. net. THE COMPLETE FOXHUNTER, 16s. net. THE COMPLETE GOLFER, 12s. 6d. net. THE COMPLETE HOCKEY-PLAYER, 10s. 6d. net. THE COMPLETE HORSEMAN, 12s. 6d. net. THE COMPLETE JUJITSUAN. Cr. 8vo. 5s. net. THE COMPLETE LAWN TENNIS PLAYER, 12s. 6d. net. THE COMPLETE MOTORIST, 10s. 6d. net. THE COMPLETE MOUNTAINEER, 16s. net. THE COMPLETE OARSMAN, 15s. net. THE COMPLETE PHOTOGRAPHER, 15s. net. THE COMPLETE RUGBY FOOTBALLER, ON THE NEW ZEALAND SYSTEM, 12s. 6d. net. THE COMPLETE SHOT, 16s. net. THE COMPLETE SWIMMER, 10s. 6d. net. THE COMPLETE YACHTSMAN, 16s. net.

The Connoisseur's Library

With numerous Illustrations. Wide Royal 8vo. 25s. net each volume

ENGLISH COLOURED BOOKS. ENGLISH FURNITURE. ETCHINGS. EUROPEAN ENAMELS. FINE BOOKS. GLASS. GOLDSMITHS' AND SILVERSMITHS' WORK. ILLUMINATED MANUSCRIPTS. IVORIES. JEWELLERY. MEZZOTINTS. MINIATURES. PORCELAIN. SEALS. WOOD SCULPTURE.

Handbooks of Theology

Demy 8vo

THE DOCTRINE OF THE INCARNATION, 15s. net. A HISTORY OF EARLY CHRISTIAN DOCTRINE, 16s. net. INTRODUCTION TO THE HISTORY OF RELIGION, 12s. 6d. net. AN INTRODUCTION TO THE HISTORY OF THE CREEDS, 12s. 6d. net. THE PHILOSOPHY OF RELIGION IN ENGLAND AND AMERICA, 12s. 6d. net. THE XXXIX ARTICLES OF THE CHURCH OF ENGLAND, 15s. net.

Health Series

Fcap. 8vo. 2s. 6d. net

THE BABY. THE CARE OF THE BODY. THE CARE OF THE TEETH. THE EYES OF OUR CHILDREN. HEALTH FOR THE MIDDLE-AGED. THE HEALTH OF A WOMAN. THE HEALTH OF THE SKIN. HOW TO LIVE LONG. THE PREVENTION OF THE COMMON COLD. STAYING THE PLAGUE. THROAT AND EAR TROUBLES. TUBERCULOSIS. THE HEALTH OF THE CHILD, 2s. net.

Leaders of Religion

Edited by H. C. BEECHING. *With Portraits*

Crown 8vo. 3s. net each volume

The Library of Devotion

Handy Editions of the great Devotional Books, well edited.
With Introductions and (where necessary) Notes

Small Pott 8vo, cloth, 3s. net and 3s. 6d. net

Little Books on Art

With many Illustrations. Demy 16mo. 5s. net each volume

Each volume consists of about 200 pages, and contains from 30 to 40 Illustrations, including a Frontispiece in Photogravure

ALBRECHT DÜRER. THE ARTS OF JAPAN.
BOOKPLATES. BOTTICELLI. BURNE-JONES.
CELLINI. CHRISTIAN SYMBOLISM. CHRIST
IN ART. CLAUDE. CONSTABLE. COROT.
EARLY ENGLISH WATER-COLOUR. ENA-
MELS. FREDERIC LEIGHTON. GEORGE
ROMNEY. GREEK ART. GREUZE AND

BOUCHER. HOLBEIN. ILLUMINATED
MANUSCRIPTS. JEWELLERY. JOHN HOPP-
NER. SIR JOSHUA REYNOLDS. MILLET.
MINIATURES. OUR LADY IN ART. RAPHAEL.
RODIN. TURNER. VANDYCK. VELAZQUEZ.
WATTS.

The Little Guides

With many Illustrations by E. H. NEW and other artists, and from photographs

Small Pott 8vo. 4s. net, 5s. net, and 6s. net

Guides to the English and Welsh Counties, and some well-known districts

The main features of these Guides are (1) a handy and charming form; (2) illustrations from photographs and by well-known artists; (3) good plans and maps; (4) an adequate but compact presentation of everything that is interesting in the natural features, history, archæology, and architecture of the town or district treated.

The Little Quarto Shakespeare

Edited by W. J. CRAIG. With Introductions and Notes

Pott 16mo. 40 Volumes. Leather, price 1s. 9d. net each volume
Cloth, 1s. 6d.

Plays

Fcap. 8vo. 3s. 6d. net

MILESTONES. Arnold Bennett and Edward Knoblock. *Ninth Edition.*

IDEAL HUSBAND, AN. Oscar Wilde. *Acting Edition.*

KISMET. Edward Knoblock. *Fourth Edition.*

TYPHOON. A Play in Four Acts. Melchior Lengyel. English Version by Laurence Irving. *Second Edition.*

WARE CASE, THE. George Pleydell.

GENERAL POST. J. E. Harold Terry. *Second Edition.*

Sports Series

Illustrated. Fcap. 8vo

ALL ABOUT FLYING, 3s. net. GOLF DO'S AND DONT'S, 2s. net. THE GOLFING SWING. 2s. 6d. net. HOW TO SWIM, 2s. net. LAWN TENNIS, 3s. net. SKATING, 3s. net.

CROSS COUNTRY SKI-ING, 5s. net. WRESTLING, 2s. net. QUICK CUTS TO GOOD GOLF, 2s. 6d. net. HOCKEY, 4s. net.

The Westminster Commentaries

General Editor, WALTER LOCK

Demy 8vo

THE ACTS OF THE APOSTLES, 16s. net. AMOS, 8s. 6d. net. I. CORINTHIANS, 8s. 6d. net. EXODUS, 15s. net. EZEKIEL, 12s. 6d. net. GENESIS, 16s. net. HEBREWS, 8s. 6d. net. ISAIAH, 16s. net. JEREMIAH,

16s. net. JOB, 8s. 6d. net. THE PASTORAL EPISTLES, 8s. 6d. net. THE PHILIPPIANS, 8s. 6d. net. ST. JAMES, 8s. 6d. net. ST. MATTHEW, 15s. net.

Methuen's Two-Shilling Library

Cheap Editions of many Popular Books
Fcap. 8vo

PART III.—A SELECTION OF WORKS OF FICTION

Bennett (Arnold)—
CLAYHANGER, 8s. net. HILDA LESSWAYS, 8s. 6d. net. THESE TWAIN. THE CARD. THE REGENT: A Five Towns Story of Adventure in London. THE PRICE OF LOVE. BURIED ALIVE. A MAN FROM THE NORTH. THE MATADOR OF THE FIVE TOWNS. WHOM GOD HATH JOINED. A GREAT MAN: A Frolic. *All 7s. 6d. net.*

Birmingham (George A.)—
SPANISH GOLD. THE SEARCH PARTY. LALAGE'S LOVERS. THE BAD TIMES. UP, THE REBELS. *All 7s. 6d. net.* INISHEENY, 8s. 6d. net.

Burroughs (Edgar Rice)—
TARZAN OF THE APES, 6s. net. THE RETURN OF TARZAN, 6s. net. THE BEASTS OF TARZAN, 6s. net. THE SON OF TARZAN, 6s. net. JUNGLE TALES OF TARZAN, 6s. net. TARZAN AND THE JEWELS OF OPAR, 6s. net. TARZAN THE UNTAMED, 7s. 6d. net. A PRINCESS OF MARS, 6s. net. THE GODS OF MARS, 6s. net. THE WARLORD OF MARS, 6s. net.

Conrad (Joseph). A SET OF SIX, 7s. 6d. net. VICTORY: An Island Tale. *Cr. 8vo. 9s. net.* THE SECRET AGENT: A Simple Tale. *Cr. 8vo. 9s. net.* UNDER WESTERN EYES. *Cr. 8vo. 9s. net.* CHANCE. *Cr. 8vo. 9s. net.*

Corelli (Marie)—
A ROMANCE OF TWO WORLDS, 7s. 6d. net. VENDETTA: or, The Story of One Forgotten, 8s. net. THELMA: A Norwegian Princess, 8s. 6d. net. ARDATH: The Story of a Dead Self, 7s. 6d. net. THE SOUL OF LILITH, 7s. 6d. net. WORMWOOD: A Drama of Paris, 8s. net. BARABBAS: A Dream of the World's Tragedy, 8s. net. THE SORROWS OF SATAN, 7s. 6d. net. THE MASTER-CHRISTIAN, 8s. 6d. net. TEMPORAL POWER: A Study in Supremacy, 6s. net. GOD'S GOOD MAN: A Simple Love Story, 8s. 6d. net. HOLY ORDERS: The Tragedy of a Quiet Life, 8s. 6d. net. THE MIGHTY ATOM, 7s. 6d. net. BOY: A Sketch, 7s. 6d. net. CAMEOS, 6s. net. THE LIFE EVERLASTING, 8s. 6d. net. THE LOVE OF LONG AGO, AND OTHER STORIES, 8s. 6d. net.

Doyle (Sir A. Conan). ROUND THE RED LAMP. *Twelfth Edition. Cr. 8vo. 7s. 6d. net.*

Hichens (Robert)—
TONGUES OF CONSCIENCE, 7s. 6d. net. FELIX: Three Years in a Life, 7s. 6d. net. THE WOMAN WITH THE FAN, 7s. 6d. net. BYEWAYS, 7s. 6d. net. THE GARDEN OF ALLAH, 8s. 6d. net. THE CALL OF THE BLOOD, 8s. 6d. net. BARBARY SHEEP, 6s. net. THE DWELLERS ON THE THRESHOLD, 7s. 6d. net. THE WAY OF AMBITION, 7s. 6d. net. IN THE WILDERNESS, 7s. 6d. net

Hope (Anthony)—
A CHANGE OF AIR. A MAN OF MARK. THE CHRONICLES OF COUNT ANTONIO. SIMON DALE. THE KING'S MIRROR. QUISANTÉ. THE DOLLY DIALOGUES. TALES OF TWO PEOPLE. A SERVANT OF THE PUBLIC. MRS. MAXON PROTESTS. A YOUNG MAN'S YEAR. BEAUMAROY HOME FROM THE WARS. *All 7s. 6d. net.*

Jacobs (W. W.)—
MANY CARGOES, 5s. net. SEA URCHINS, 5s. net and 3s. 6d. net. A MASTER OF CRAFT, 5s. net. LIGHT FREIGHTS, 5s. net. THE SKIPPER'S WOOING, 5s. net. AT SUN-WICH PORT, 5s. net. DIALSTONE LANE, 5s. net. ODD CRAFT, 5s. net. THE LADY OF THE BARGE, 5s. net. SALTHAVEN, 5s. net. SAILORS' KNOTS, 5s. net. SHORT CRUISES, 6s. net.

London (Jack). WHITE FANG. *Ninth Edition. Cr. 8vo. 7s. 6d. net.*

Lucas (E. V.)—
LISTENER'S LURE: An Oblique Narration, 6s. net. OVER BEMERTON'S: An Easy-going Chronicle, 6s. net. MR. INGLESIDE, 6s. net. LONDON LAVENDER, 6s. net. LANDMARKS, 7s. 6d. net. THE VERMILION BOX, 7s. 6d. net. VERENA IN THE MIDST, 8s. 6d. net.

McKenna (Stephen)—
SONIA: Between Two Worlds, 8s. net. NINETY-SIX HOURS' LEAVE, 7s. 6d. net. THE SIXTH SENSE, 6s. net. MIDAS & SON, 8s. net.

Malet (Lucas)—
THE HISTORY OF SIR RICHARD CALMADY: A Romance. THE CARISSIMA. THE GATELESS BARRIER. DEADHAM HARD. *All 7s. 6d. net.* THE WAGES OF SIN. 8s. net.

Mason (A. E. W.). CLEMENTINA. Illustrated. *Ninth Edition. Cr. 8vo. 7s. 6d. net.*

Maxwell (W. B.)—
VIVIEN. THE GUARDED FLAME. ODD LENGTHS. HILL RISE. THE REST CURE. *All 7s. 6d. net.*

Oxenham (John)—
A WEAVER OF WEBS. PROFIT AND LOSS. THE SONG OF HYACINTH, and Other Stories. LAURISTONS. THE COIL OF CARNE. THE QUEST OF THE GOLDEN ROSE. MARY ALL-ALONE. BROKEN SHACKLES. "1914." *All 7s. 6d. net.*

Parker (Gilbert)—
PIERRE AND HIS PEOPLE. MRS. FALCHION. THE TRANSLATION OF A SAVAGE. WHEN VALMOND CAME TO PONTIAC: The Story of a Lost Napoleon. AN ADVENTURER OF THE NORTH: The Last Adventures of 'Pretty Pierre.' THE SEATS OF THE MIGHTY. THE BATTLE OF THE STRONG: A Romance of Two Kingdoms. THE POMP OF THE LAVILETTES. NORTHERN LIGHTS. *All 7s. 6d. net.*

Phillpotts (Eden)—
CHILDREN OF THE MIST. SONS OF THE MORNING. THE RIVER. THE AMERICAN PRISONER. DEMETER'S DAUGHTER. THE HUMAN BOY AND THE WAR. *All 7s. 6d. net.*

Ridge (W. Pett)—
A SON OF THE STATE, 7s. 6d. net. THE REMINGTON SENTENCE, 7s. 6d. net. MADAME PRINCE, 7s. 6d. net. TOP SPEED, 7s. 6d. net. SPECIAL PERFORMANCES, 6s. net. THE BUSTLING HOURS, 7s. 6d. net.

Rohmer (Sax)—
THE DEVIL DOCTOR. THE SI-FAN MYSTERIES. TALES OF SECRET EGYPT. THE ORCHARD OF TEARS. THE GOLDEN SCORPION. *All 7s. 6d. net.*

Swinnerton (F.). SHOPS AND HOUSES. *Third Edition. Cr. 8vo. 7s. 6d. net.*

SEPTEMBER. *Third Edition. Cr. 8vo. 7s. 6d. net.*

THE HAPPY FAMILY. *Second Edition. 7s. 6d. net.*

ON THE STAIRCASE. *Third Edition. 7s. 6d. net.*

Wells (H. G.). BEALBY. *Fourth Edition. Cr. 8vo. 7s. 6d. net.*

Williamson (C. N. and A. M.)—
THE LIGHTNING CONDUCTOR: The Strange Adventures of a Motor Car. LADY BETTY ACROSS THE WATER. SCARLET RUNNER. LORD LOVELAND DISCOVERS AMERICA. THE GUESTS OF HERCULES. IT HAPPENED IN EGYPT. A SOLDIER OF THE LEGION. THE SHOP GIRL. THE LIGHTNING CON-DUCTRESS. SECRET HISTORY. THE LOVE PIRATE. *All 7s. 6d. net.* CRUCIFIX CORNER. 6s. net.

Methuen's Two-Shilling Novels

Cheap Editions of many of the most Popular Novels of the day

Write for Complete List

Fcap. 8vo

THE PSYCHOLOGY OF MEDICINE